Quiet Reflections: Wisdom and Strategies for Midlife Solitude

ETTIE O'BRYAN

ISBN: 9798304791953

ISBN: 9798304791953

DEDICATION

To the Women Who Walk This Path and to Future Generations: This book is dedicated to all those who courageously navigate the journey of midlife solitude. May you find strength, wisdom, and peace within these pages, and discover the power to embrace the next chapter of your life with grace and empowerment.

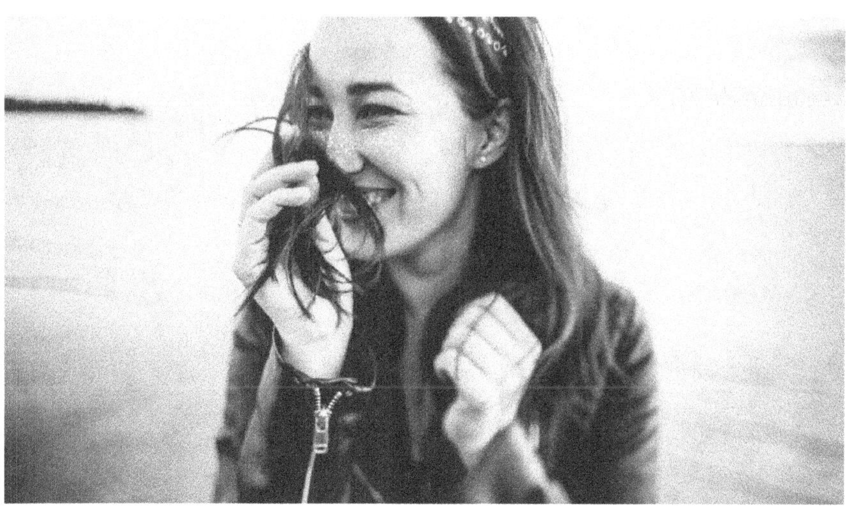

ACKNOWLEDGMENTS

This book is a testament to the strength and courage of women and readers alike, whose stories and journeys have deeply inspired me.

To the incredible women who shared their personal experiences, your bravery and candour have brought this work to life in ways I could never have imagined. Your voices echo through these pages, offering wisdom, resilience, and hope to all who encounter them.

To the readers who have embarked on this journey, thank you for your openness and curiosity. Your willingness to explore the complexities of midlife solitude is both humbling and inspiring. May these words empower you to embrace your path with grace and transformation, as you embody the beauty of renewal and growth.

PREFACE

As a mental health counsellor, my journey into specializing in menopause mental health began with my own experience navigating this transformative stage of life. Like many women, I was confronted with the profound changes that menopause brings — both physically and emotionally. It was during this personal journey that I realized just how many women in midlife were grappling with similar challenges, often in solitude and silence.

This shared experience sparked my passion to explore the often-unspoken realm of midlife solitude and its impact on mental health. Through my work, I have had the privilege of supporting many women as they navigate the complexities of midlife and menopause. These experiences have shaped the foundation of "Quiet Reflections: Wisdom and Strategies for Midlife Solitude."

This book is a culmination of my professional insights and personal journey. It delves deep into the psychological landscape of loneliness, offering research-based strategies tailored specifically for women experiencing the profound changes of menopause. With compassion and expertise, it uncovers the hidden strengths within solitude, inviting readers to redefine their identities and embrace newfound resilience.

As you turn these pages, you will discover the power of purpose and the art of building meaningful connections, all while nurturing holistic health in both body and mind. Inspired by the ancient proverb, "Solitude is the furnace of transformation," this book serves as a beacon of hope and empowerment for those ready to embrace the next chapter of life with grace and wisdom.

Whether you are seeking solace, inspiration, or a deeper understanding of self, "Quiet Reflections" offers a sanctuary of knowledge and strategies to thrive in the beauty of midlife solitude. It is my hope that this book will guide you on your own path of self-discovery and renewal, empowering you to embrace the unique journey of midlife with courage and clarity.

May these reflections provide you with strength and wisdom, serving as a catalyst for your personal transformation, just as they have in my own life and in the lives of countless others.

CONTENTS

INTRODUCTION

As the sun dipped below the horizon, casting a golden hue over the quiet lake, Maria sat on her porch, enveloped by the serene solitude of the evening. It was in these moments, away from the bustling world, that she found herself reflecting on life's transitions — particularly, the unexpected quiet that had settled in as she traversed the path of midlife. For Maria, and many women like her, this period of life brought with it a profound sense of solitude, a silence that was both daunting and liberating.

Welcome to 'Quiet Reflections: Wisdom and Strategies for Midlife Solitude,' a book crafted to guide you through this significant phase with understanding and empowerment. This introduction aims to provide a sweeping overview of the journey ahead, introducing you to the rich tapestry of themes and ideas woven throughout the book.

The purpose of this book is twofold: to illuminate the complex emotional and psychological landscape of midlife solitude and to offer practical wisdom and strategies for embracing this time as an opportunity for growth and self-discovery. By exploring the intersection of psychological research on loneliness and the unique experiences of women undergoing menopause, this book seeks to validate and support those navigating these uncharted waters.

Key themes include the silent transition into midlife, the science of loneliness, the empowerment found in solitude, and the redefinition of identity. The book also delves into building resilience, creating connections, and discovering purpose, all while emphasizing the importance of holistic health.

Structured into ten insightful chapters, each section builds upon the last, leading you through a journey of transformation. From understanding the initial silence to embracing the next life chapter, the book offers a roadmap of reflection and action.

While this book focuses primarily on women over 50 experiencing menopause, its insights hold universal relevance for anyone encountering solitude in midlife. However, it is not exhaustive; rather, it serves as a starting point for deeper exploration and personal growth. The significance of 'Quiet Reflections' lies in its ability to transform solitude from a source of loneliness into a wellspring of strength and self-awareness. It contributes to the field by intertwining contemporary psychological insights with the timeless wisdom of embracing life's quieter moments.

In summary, this introduction sets the stage for a transformative journey, beckoning you to explore the richness of midlife solitude and the incredible potential it holds. Let Maria's story be a reminder that within the silence, there lies an opportunity for profound discovery and renewal.

CHAPTER 1

The Silent Transition: Understanding Midlife Solitude

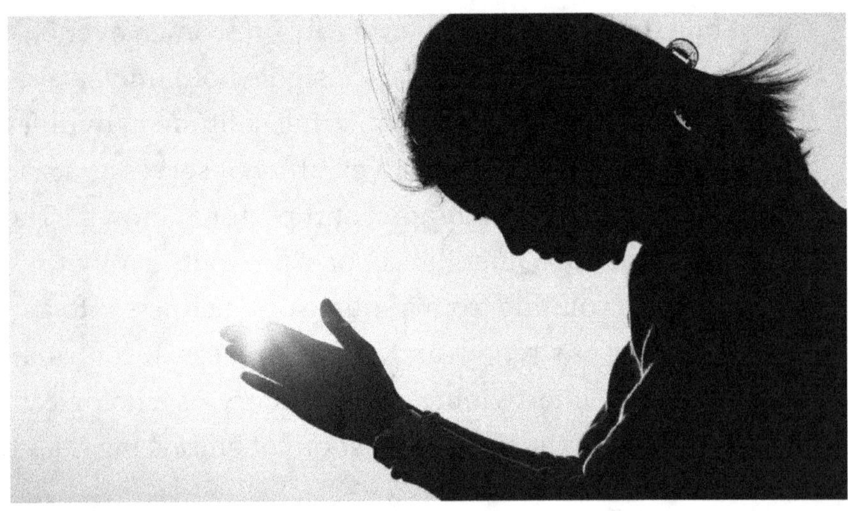

In the quiet corridors of midlife, many women find themselves navigating a complex landscape of emotions and experiences that often remain unspoken. This period, marked by the profound physical and emotional transition of menopause, can sometimes feel like a whisper, a silent transition into a new phase of life. It is in this hushed moment that solitude can become both a companion and a teacher, gently urging us to listen more intently to the rhythms of our own hearts. As the renowned proverb suggests, 'The quieter you become, the more you can hear.' These words resonate deeply within the context of midlife solitude, inviting women to embrace the silence as a fertile ground for introspection and growth.

Recent psychological research has shed light on the phenomenon of loneliness, particularly among women over 50. Studies indicate that this demographic is increasingly susceptible to feelings of isolation, often exacerbated by the physiological and emotional changes accompanying menopause. This natural transition, while a universal experience, can significantly impact a woman's emotional well-being, sometimes leading to heightened feelings of loneliness and disconnection.

Yet, within this solitude lies an opportunity for profound transformation. The silence of midlife offers a unique space for reflection, a chance to reassess one's identity and redefine personal goals. It is a period ripe with potential for self-discovery, allowing women to peel back the layers of their past and explore the depths of their true selves. In this quietude, there exists a remarkable opportunity to hear the whispers of one's own soul, to understand the unspoken needs and desires that have been overshadowed by the noise of daily life.

The intersection of menopause and solitude can also serve as a powerful catalyst for personal growth. As women confront the changes occurring within their bodies, they may find themselves questioning their roles, relationships, and priorities. This introspective journey, though initially daunting, can lead to a newfound sense of clarity and purpose. By embracing the silence, women can learn to listen to their inner wisdom, nurturing a deeper understanding of who they are and what they truly value.

Moreover, this chapter will delve into the intriguing psychological research that highlights the paradoxical nature of loneliness. While often viewed as a negative emotion, loneliness can also be a driving force for positive change. It can inspire creativity, foster resilience, and encourage the formation of meaningful connections with others. By understanding the science behind loneliness, women can begin to see solitude not as a barrier, but as a bridge to a richer, more fulfilling life.

In the journey through midlife solitude, it is crucial to recognize the hidden strengths that lie within this quiet transformation. The silence is not an empty void, but a space filled with potential and possibility. It is an invitation to listen more closely, to hear the truths that have long been buried beneath the surface. As we explore the silent transition into midlife solitude, we will uncover the ways in which this experience can serve as a powerful source of empowerment and renewal. Together, we will embark on a journey of understanding, reflection, and growth, embracing the wisdom that comes with listening deeply to the quiet echoes of our hearts.

1.1 The Silent Transition: Unveiling the Layers of Loneliness

As we embark on the journey of midlife, a profound transformation often begins to take shape, one that whispers quietly yet insistently. This is the silent transition into solitude—a phase marked by a reawakening of self-awareness, a re-evaluation of purpose, and, for many women over 50, an encounter with the often-misunderstood phenomenon of loneliness. In this section, we delve into the intricate tapestry of psychological research that illuminates the prevalence and impact of loneliness among midlife women.

Unravelling Loneliness: A Silent Epidemic

Loneliness, as elusive as it may seem, is a significant psychological experience, particularly prevalent among women entering their midlife years. According to recent studies, nearly 60% of women over the age of 50 report experiencing feelings of loneliness. This statistic, however, only scratches the surface of a more complex emotional landscape. Loneliness in midlife is not merely a lack of social connections but a deeper sense of disconnection from oneself and the surrounding world.

One such study conducted by the University of California, San Francisco, highlights that loneliness is not synonymous with being alone. Instead, it is an emotional state characterized by a perceived gap between desired and actual social interaction. For women transitioning through menopause, this gap can widen due to a confluence of factors—changing family dynamics, retirement, and the loss of societal roles that once defined their identity.

The Psychological Landscape: Understanding the Impact

The psychological impact of loneliness during midlife is profound. It has been linked to an array of mental health challenges, including depression, anxiety, and a heightened risk of cognitive decline. Research from Brigham Young University suggests that loneliness can be as detrimental to health as smoking 15 cigarettes a day. This startling comparison underscores the importance of addressing loneliness as a critical health issue.

For women in midlife, the experience of loneliness can be exacerbated by the hormonal fluctuations of menopause. The decline of oestrogen levels affects mood regulation, often leading to increased irritability and feelings of sadness. This hormonal shift, coupled with societal expectations and personal transitions, creates a perfect storm that can magnify the sense of isolation.

The Intersection of Loneliness and Identity

As women navigate the complexities of midlife, a pivotal question arises: "Who am I now?" This period of transition often prompts a re-examination of identity, as previous roles and responsibilities evolve. The loneliness experienced is not just an emotional state but a reflection of the struggle to redefine oneself in the absence of familiar markers.

In her seminal work, Brené Brown, a renowned researcher on vulnerability and courage, emphasizes that loneliness is, at its core, the absence of connection. For women over 50, reestablishing a sense of connection—both with themselves and others—is essential to overcoming loneliness. This process involves embracing vulnerability and acknowledging the inherent strength in seeking new paths of self-discovery.

The Wisdom of Solitude: Embracing the Journey

While loneliness can be a formidable adversary, it also holds the potential for profound personal growth. In the words of the ancient philosopher Lao Tzu, "Knowing others is intelligence; knowing yourself is true wisdom." Embracing solitude as a transformative journey can empower women to delve deeper into self-awareness and cultivate resilience.

Solitude provides a unique opportunity for introspection and self-reflection, allowing women to rediscover passions, set new goals, and forge a renewed sense of purpose. This period of quiet reflection can be harnessed to nurture creativity, foster personal development, and establish meaningful connections with the self.

Strategies for Navigating Loneliness

To navigate the silent transition of midlife solitude, women can employ a variety of strategies that foster connection and resilience. Engaging in community activities, pursuing hobbies, and volunteering are powerful ways to combat loneliness and enhance social ties. Additionally, seeking support groups or therapy can provide a safe space to explore emotions and develop coping mechanisms.

Mindfulness practices, such as meditation and journaling, offer tools for cultivating self-awareness and managing stress. By prioritizing self-care and embracing the present moment, women can build emotional resilience and foster a deeper connection with themselves.

Conclusion: A Beacon of Hope and Transformation

As we conclude this exploration of midlife loneliness, it is essential to recognize that solitude, while challenging, is also a fertile ground for transformation. By reframing loneliness as an invitation to reconnect with oneself and others, women can embark on a journey of empowerment, resilience, and enduring wisdom.

In embracing the silent transition, women over 50 can redefine their narrative, celebrating the beauty of midlife solitude as a catalyst for personal growth and renewal. By weaving the threads of psychological research with the timeless wisdom of self-discovery, we illuminate a path to thriving in the serenity of solitude, creating a legacy of strength for future generations.

1.2 The Natural Shift: Embracing Change

As we delve deeper into the subject of midlife solitude, it's imperative to first acknowledge the natural transition that is menopause and its profound impact on emotional well-being. Menopause is a biological milestone that marks the end of a woman's reproductive years, typically occurring between the ages of 45 and 55. This phase is not just a physical transformation but a complex interplay of hormonal changes that influence emotional and psychological health.

The Biological Underpinnings

Menopause is characterized by a decrease in ovarian production of oestrogen and progesterone, the hormones responsible for regulating the menstrual cycle. This hormonal shift can lead to a variety of symptoms, including hot flashes, night sweats, sleep disturbances, and mood swings. The fluctuating hormone levels can also affect neurotransmitters in the brain, such as serotonin and dopamine, which are closely linked to mood regulation. This biological upheaval can contribute to feelings of loneliness and isolation, further complicating the emotional landscape of midlife.

Psychological Perspectives

From a psychological standpoint, menopause can be perceived as a period of loss — the loss of fertility, the end of a significant life stage, and sometimes, the reduction of perceived feminine identity. This can trigger a re-evaluation of self-worth and purpose, leading to introspection and, occasionally, a sense of solitude. However, solitude during this time can be both a challenge and an opportunity for personal growth.

The Role of Loneliness

Recent psychological research has highlighted the link between menopause and increased feelings of loneliness. A study published in the journal 'Menopause' found that women experiencing menopausal symptoms reported higher levels of loneliness compared to their pre-menopausal counterparts. The study suggests that the physical symptoms of menopause can contribute to withdrawal from social activities, exacerbating feelings of isolation. It is crucial to recognize this transition as a natural process and not a solitary journey.

Solitude as a Catalyst for Self-Discovery

Solitude in midlife, especially during menopause, can serve as a powerful catalyst for self-discovery. Instead of perceiving this solitude as loneliness, it can be reframed as an opportunity for introspection and growth. The quiet moments that accompany this life stage allow for a deep dive into personal passions, interests, and long-forgotten dreams. In the words of the renowned poet Rainer Maria Rilke, "The only journey is the journey within."

Redefining Identity

Menopause presents an opportunity to redefine one's identity beyond societal and familial roles. It is a time to explore new facets of oneself that may have been neglected while fulfilling other responsibilities. This redefinition can lead to a more authentic sense of self, rooted in individual values and desires rather than external expectations.

The Wisdom of Solitude

The proverb "Solitude is the furnace of transformation" aptly captures the essence of this life phase. In solitude, one finds the space to reflect, heal, and ultimately transform. This period of introspection can lead to a renewed sense of purpose and the courage to pursue new directions in life.

Strategies for Navigating Emotional Well-being

Mindfulness and Meditation

Incorporating mindfulness and meditation practices into daily life can help manage the emotional fluctuations associated with menopause. These practices promote self-awareness and emotional regulation, allowing for a more balanced approach to the challenges of this transition.

Building Resilience

Building resilience is crucial in navigating the emotional waves of menopause. Developing coping strategies, such as maintaining strong social connections and engaging in regular physical activity, can enhance emotional well-being. Resilience empowers individuals to adapt positively to change, fostering a sense of control and empowerment.

Seeking Professional Support

It is important to recognize when professional support is needed. Therapy or counselling can provide a safe space to explore emotions, develop coping mechanisms, and receive validation for the experiences unique to this life stage. Seeking support is a sign of strength and a proactive step toward emotional well-being.

Conclusion: Embracing the Journey

The silent transition of menopause is a multifaceted journey that encompasses physical, emotional, and psychological transformations. By understanding the natural shift that occurs during this time, women can better navigate the complexities of midlife solitude. Embracing this transition as an opportunity for self-discovery and personal growth can lead to a more fulfilling and empowered life. As you move forward on this journey, remember that solitude is not synonymous with loneliness but a sacred space for transformation and renewal.

1.3 Whispers of Introspection: The Power of Listening to Oneself

The Quiet Revolution: Listening to the Heart

In the bustling noise of modern life, the art of listening often becomes lost amidst the clamour of obligations and expectations. Yet, in the serenity of solitude, there lies an opportunity to turn inward and truly listen to one's own heart. The proverb 'The quieter you become, the more you can hear' holds profound wisdom for those navigating the silent transition of midlife solitude. As women enter this transformative phase, marked by the onset of menopause and the myriad changes it brings, embracing quietude allows for a deepened understanding of personal desires and needs.

Midlife is often a time of reflection and reassessment. The roles and responsibilities that once defined us may shift, leaving a void that is both unsettling and liberating. In this space, listening to our innermost thoughts and emotions can unveil long-buried passions and unfulfilled dreams. It's a gentle revolution, a call to rediscover the essence of who we are beyond societal labels and familial roles.

Embracing the Science: Insights into Loneliness and Self-Discovery

Psychological research underscores the transformative power of solitude. Studies reveal that periods of intentional solitude can enhance self-awareness and foster personal growth. Yet, the line between solitude and loneliness is delicate. Loneliness, particularly in midlife, can emerge as a daunting adversary, exacerbated by the hormonal fluctuations and emotional upheavals of menopause.

Research conducted by neuroscientists at the University of Chicago has shown that loneliness activates neural pathways in the brain associated with pain. This insight highlights the importance of addressing feelings of isolation with compassion and understanding. For women over 50, acknowledging these emotions is crucial. Solitude should not be equated with loneliness but viewed as a fertile ground for introspection and self-renewal.

As women embrace solitude, they can harness its potential to explore their identities and redefine their life's purpose. This process requires embracing the quiet, listening to the whispers of introspection, and allowing them to guide the journey toward self-discovery.

Menopause and the Midlife Metamorphosis

Menopause, often referred to as the 'change of life,' is a pivotal period in a woman's journey. It ushers in a metamorphosis, not just biologically but emotionally and psychologically. The hormonal shifts can lead to mood swings, anxiety, and feelings of vulnerability. However, within these challenges lie opportunities for profound transformation.

In embracing the solitude of menopause, women can cultivate a deeper understanding of their evolving selves. The transition is an invitation to shed old skins and embrace new identities. With quiet introspection, they can navigate the emotional waves of menopause with resilience and grace. The silence becomes a sanctuary where they can reflect on past experiences, glean lessons, and craft a vision for the future.

The Inner Dialogue: Cultivating Compassion and Self-Acceptance

Listening to oneself involves engaging in an inner dialogue that is both honest and compassionate. It's about recognizing and validating one's emotions without judgment. For many women, midlife marks a time when self-compassion becomes essential. The pressures of perfectionism and societal expectations can be heavy burdens, but solitude offers the space to release these weights.

By fostering self-acceptance, women can begin to heal and nurture their inner selves. This process involves acknowledging past wounds, forgiving oneself for perceived shortcomings, and embracing the imperfect beauty of one's journey. The quietude of solitude provides a nurturing environment for this inner work, allowing women to emerge with renewed strength and confidence.

Navigating the Solitude: Practical Strategies for Self-Reflection

To fully embrace the solitude of midlife, practical strategies can be employed to facilitate self-reflection and introspection. Journaling is a powerful tool that allows women to articulate their thoughts and emotions. Writing provides a safe space to explore fears, aspirations, and desires, offering clarity and insight.

Mindfulness practices, such as meditation and deep breathing exercises, can also aid in quieting the mind and tuning into one's inner voice. These practices encourage presence and awareness, helping women cultivate a deeper connection with themselves. By setting aside time each day for mindfulness, women can create a sacred space for introspection amidst the chaos of daily life.

The Wisdom of Solitude: Embracing the Journey

The journey of midlife solitude is one of profound wisdom and transformation. It's a time to explore the depths of one's being and embrace the quiet strength within. As women navigate this transition, they are called to listen to their hearts and honour the whispers of introspection.

The proverb 'The quieter you become, the more you can hear' serves as a guiding light, reminding women of the power of silence and self-discovery. In embracing solitude, they embark on a journey of empowerment and renewal, discovering the beauty of their authentic selves and the limitless potential within.

By cultivating a practice of introspection, women can redefine midlife not as a time of decline but as a vibrant new chapter filled with possibility and purpose. This silent transition is a testament to the resilience and strength of the human spirit, a celebration of the wisdom that comes with embracing the quietude of solitude.

1.4 Embracing the Silence: A Path to Self-Discovery

As we conclude our journey through the silent transition of midlife solitude, it's essential to recognize that this period, though challenging, offers profound opportunities for growth and understanding. The psychological research highlights the prevalence of loneliness among women over 50, reminding us that we are not alone in experiencing these emotions. Acknowledging this commonality can be the first step in forging connections and seeking support. Furthermore, the natural transition of menopause is not just a biological change but also a catalyst for emotional transformation. Understanding its impact on our well-being allows us to approach this phase with compassion and self-awareness.

The proverb, 'The quieter you become, the more you can hear,' serves as a guiding principle in this chapter. It invites us to embrace introspection, to listen to the whispers of our inner selves, often drowned out by the noise of daily life. In solitude, we find the space to reflect, to heal, and to rediscover our passions and purpose.

Key takeaways from this chapter include recognizing loneliness as a shared experience and leveraging it to build meaningful connections. Accept the menopausal transition as a time to nurture emotional health, and, most importantly, utilize solitude as a powerful tool for introspection. Moving forward, I encourage you to carve out moments of silence in your life, to listen to the wisdom within, and to allow it to guide your path to self-discovery and fulfilment. This journey is not about escaping solitude but embracing it as a transformative companion.

Chapter 1: Reflection Time

- Reflect on a time when you felt lonely. How did you cope with it, and what did you learn from that experience?
- How has your understanding of solitude and loneliness evolved over time, especially as you approach or experience midlife?
- In what ways can embracing solitude lead to personal growth and introspection for you?

CHAPTER 2

The Science of Loneliness: A Psychological Perspective

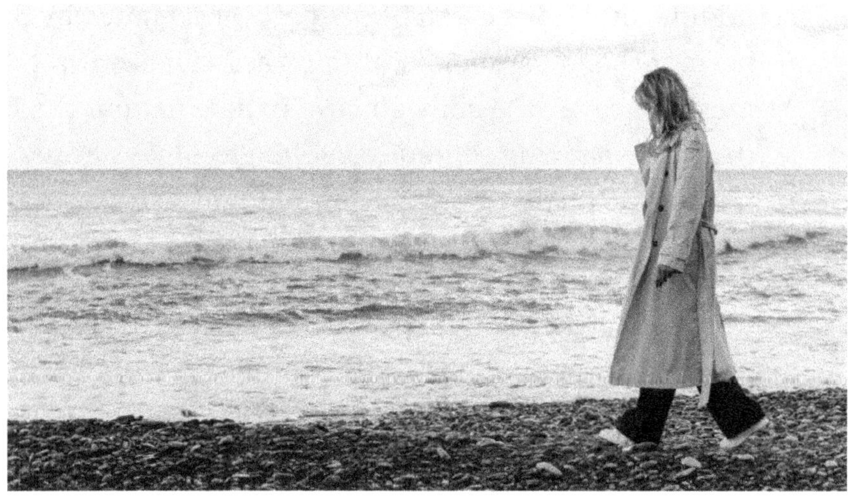

In a world that is perpetually connected, the paradox of loneliness remains a profound enigma, particularly for women navigating the transformative journey of menopause. As we delve into the second chapter of 'Quiet Reflections: Wisdom and Strategies for Midlife Solitude,' we shift our focus to unravel the intricate science of loneliness, examining its psychological underpinnings and its significant impact on both mental and physical health. This chapter serves as a crucial bridge between understanding the silent transition of midlife solitude and embracing the transformative power of solitude itself.

Loneliness, as research consistently illustrates, is not just an emotional experience but a state that can significantly affect our overall well-being. Studies have shown that chronic loneliness can lead to increased levels of stress, anxiety, and depression, as well as a higher risk of cardiovascular diseases and weakened immune responses. For women in midlife, these effects can be further compounded by the hormonal and psychological shifts associated with menopause. As the body adjusts to these natural changes, the accompanying solitude can often feel like a heavy burden rather than an opportunity for growth.

The psychological perspective on loneliness reveals that it is deeply intertwined with our perceptions of social connectedness and self-worth. Mother Teresa poignantly encapsulated this sentiment when she observed, 'Loneliness and the feeling of being unwanted is the most terrible poverty.' Her words remind us that loneliness is not just about being alone but about feeling isolated, undervalued, and unseen. In the context of menopause, these feelings can be exacerbated by societal shifts and personal life events, such as children leaving home, retirement, or changes in marital status, which can alter a woman's social environment and support systems.

As we explore the psychological dimensions of loneliness, it is essential to consider how societal changes have influenced the experience of solitude during menopause. Historically, menopause has been shrouded in silence, often dismissed or stigmatized. However, recent societal shifts towards increased awareness and open dialogue have begun to reshape this narrative, offering women the opportunity to redefine their midlife experiences. Despite these advancements, the challenge remains to navigate the personal and societal expectations that can contribute to feelings of loneliness during this period.

This chapter seeks to illuminate the hidden dynamics of loneliness, providing a comprehensive understanding of its psychological foundations. By examining groundbreaking studies and expert insights, we aim to equip readers with the knowledge needed to recognize and address loneliness in their own lives. As we journey through the pages ahead, we will uncover the strategies and wisdom necessary to transform loneliness from a source of despair into a catalyst for personal growth and resilience.

In this exploration, we invite readers to reflect on their own experiences and perceptions of loneliness. Through understanding the science behind this complex emotion, we hope to empower women to embrace their solitude with newfound clarity and confidence. As we delve deeper into the psychological landscape of loneliness, let us hold onto the wisdom that while loneliness may feel like an insurmountable poverty, it also offers the potential for profound personal transformation and connection with one's innermost self.

Join us as we embark on this enlightening journey, where the science of loneliness becomes a guiding light, illuminating the path towards a richer, more fulfilled experience of midlife solitude.

2.1 Loneliness: The Unseen Shadow

Introduction: The Silent Epidemic

In the quiet recesses of our daily lives, loneliness lurks like an unseen shadow, often unnoticed but profoundly impactful. While it is an experience that can affect people at any stage of life, its presence becomes particularly pronounced during midlife—a period marked by significant transitions such as menopause. This chapter delves into the psychological underpinnings of loneliness, examining its far-reaching effects on both mental and physical health, and exploring how it specifically impacts women over 50.

The Psychological Impact of Loneliness

Loneliness is not merely a state of mind; it is a complex emotional experience that has been extensively studied in psychological research. According to a seminal study by psychologist John Cacioppo, loneliness can trigger a cascade of psychological responses that amplify feelings of sadness, depression, and anxiety. This emotional turmoil is particularly pronounced during midlife, as women face the dual challenges of navigating menopause and redefining their identities.

The psychological impact of loneliness is deeply intertwined with self-perception. Women over 50 often find themselves grappling with a sense of invisibility in a society that prioritizes youth. This perceived lack of relevance can exacerbate feelings of isolation, leading to a vicious cycle where loneliness fuels negative self-perception, and negative self-perception, in turn, deepens loneliness.

Loneliness and Physical Health: The Hidden Toll

Beyond its psychological footprint, loneliness exacts a significant toll on physical health. Research conducted by the University of California, San Francisco, found that chronic loneliness increases the risk of cardiovascular diseases, inflammation, and even mortality. This is attributed to the body's stress response, which is activated by feelings of isolation and leads to increased production of stress hormones like cortisol.

For women in midlife, the physiological changes accompanying menopause can amplify the physical effects of loneliness. As oestrogen levels decline, women may experience heightened anxiety and depression, which, when coupled with loneliness, can lead to detrimental health outcomes such as heart disease and weakened immune function.

The Intersection of Loneliness and Menopause

The experience of menopause can be a solitary journey, often fraught with misunderstandings and societal taboos. This life stage represents a significant transition, as women redefine their roles and cope with the physical changes that accompany the end of their reproductive years. The intersection of loneliness and menopause can create a perfect storm of emotional and physical challenges.

A study published in the journal Menopause highlights the increased risk of depressive symptoms in postmenopausal women who report feeling lonely. The hormonal fluctuations during menopause can exacerbate mood swings, while the sense of social isolation can intensify these emotions. This research underscores the importance of addressing loneliness as a critical component of menopausal care.

Coping Strategies: Finding Light in the Shadows

Despite the daunting challenges posed by loneliness, there are effective strategies that women can adopt to mitigate its effects. Cognitive-behavioural therapy (CBT) has proven to be a powerful tool in helping individuals reframe negative thought patterns and develop healthier coping mechanisms. For women navigating midlife solitude, CBT can foster resilience and empower them to embrace life changes with a positive outlook.

Additionally, mindfulness practices such as meditation and yoga can provide solace and reduce stress. These practices encourage individuals to focus on the present moment, fostering a sense of inner peace that can counteract the feelings of isolation. For women experiencing menopause, engaging in regular physical activity can also alleviate symptoms such as mood swings and hot flashes, while promoting overall well-being.

Building Connections: The Antidote to Loneliness

One of the most effective ways to combat loneliness is to build meaningful social connections. Research has shown that maintaining strong social ties can significantly reduce the health risks associated with loneliness. For women in midlife, this may involve rekindling old friendships, joining community groups, or participating in support networks specifically tailored for menopausal women.

A study conducted by the Harvard Women's Health Watch found that women who maintain close relationships with friends and family report higher levels of happiness and lower levels of stress. These connections provide emotional support and a sense of belonging that can counteract the isolating effects of loneliness.

Proverbial Wisdom: "A Shared Burden is a Lighter Load"

As women navigate the complexities of loneliness and menopause, the wisdom encapsulated in the proverb "A shared burden is a lighter load" becomes particularly poignant. By reaching out and sharing their experiences with others, women can lighten their emotional load and find strength in solidarity. This sense of community serves as a powerful reminder that they are not alone in their journey.

Conclusion: Embracing Solitude's Potential

While loneliness can cast a long shadow, it is also an opportunity for profound personal growth and transformation. By understanding the psychological and physical effects of loneliness, women can take proactive steps to embrace solitude as a source of strength and resilience. Through self-discovery and connection, they can redefine their identities and find purpose in this new chapter of life.

In 'Quiet Reflections,' we invite you to turn toward the light, to seek wisdom in solitude, and to uncover the hidden strengths that lie within. As you embrace the journey of midlife solitude, may you find solace in the knowledge that you are capable of thriving in this beautiful, transformative period of life.

2.2 The Ripple Effect: Navigating the Complexities of Loneliness During Menopause

In the tapestry of a woman's life, midlife often emerges as a profound juncture characterized by a cascade of transformations, both physical and emotional. Menopause, a natural biological process, is one such transition. While it marks the end of reproductive years, it also heralds a time of introspection and solitude. As women step into this phase, societal changes and personal life events can significantly amplify feelings of loneliness. Understanding these dynamics is crucial to embracing solitude as a catalyst for growth and self-discovery.

The Societal Shifts: A Changing Landscape

In contemporary society, the roles and expectations surrounding women have evolved dramatically over the decades. Women today often juggle multiple responsibilities, from nurturing families to advancing careers. As they enter midlife, however, societal perceptions can shift. The ageist stereotypes that permeate many cultures subtly suggest that older women are less relevant or impactful. This can lead to feelings of invisibility and isolation, exacerbating loneliness during menopause.

Moreover, the societal emphasis on youth and beauty can affect self-esteem and self-worth. Women may feel pressured to maintain an image that aligns with societal ideals, leading to a dissonance between their internal and external realities. This tension can foster a sense of loneliness as they grapple with the fading echoes of roles and identities that once defined them.

Personal Life Events: Unravelling the Threads of Connection

The midlife transition often coincides with significant personal life events that can accentuate loneliness. The 'empty nest' syndrome, for instance, is a poignant example. As children grow up and leave the family home, women may experience a void that once was filled with the daily rhythms of parenting. This transition can leave them questioning their purpose and longing for the connections that sustained them.

Simultaneously, midlife can usher in changes in marital or partnership dynamics. Relationships may evolve, and in some cases, dissolve. Divorce or the death of a partner can plunge individuals into profound solitude, challenging them to navigate new emotional terrains. The loss of a lifelong companion or confidante can intensify feelings of isolation, leaving women to rebuild their social networks and redefine their support systems.

The Biological Underpinnings: Hormonal Changes and Emotional Waves

Biologically, menopause is marked by a decline in oestrogen and progesterone levels, which can significantly impact mood and emotional well-being. Hormonal fluctuations can lead to symptoms such as irritability, anxiety, and depression, all of which can contribute to a heightened sense of loneliness. The psychological impact of these changes is profound, often leading women to question their mental health and emotional resilience.

Research has shown that loneliness can have tangible effects on the brain. Studies suggest that prolonged loneliness can alter neural pathways, affecting cognitive function and increasing the risk of depression. Understanding the interplay between hormonal changes and emotional health is vital for women navigating the complexities of midlife solitude.

The Cultural Narrative: Redefining Solitude and Connection

In many cultures, solitude is often perceived negatively, equated with loneliness and social isolation. However, reframing solitude as a space for reflection and growth can be empowering. Women in midlife are presented with an opportunity to redefine their narratives, embracing solitude as a time to reconnect with their inner selves and explore new dimensions of identity.

This cultural shift requires a conscious effort to challenge the traditional views of aging and femininity. By embracing solitude, women can cultivate a deeper understanding of their aspirations, values, and passions. This period of introspection can foster resilience, allowing them to emerge stronger and more self-assured.

Strategies for Embracing Solitude: Practical Approaches

To effectively navigate the loneliness that may accompany menopause, women can adopt strategies that foster connection and self-awareness. Mindfulness practices, such as meditation and yoga, offer a pathway to inner peace and self-discovery. These practices encourage individuals to be present in the moment, cultivating an awareness of their thoughts and emotions.

Engaging in creative pursuits, whether through art, music, or writing, can also serve as an outlet for expression and connection. Creativity allows women to tap into their inner worlds, fostering a sense of purpose and fulfilment. Additionally, volunteering and community involvement can provide opportunities for meaningful interactions, strengthening social ties and combating loneliness.

A Proverb's Wisdom: Finding Strength in Solitude

Reflecting on the ancient proverb, 'Solitude is the furnace of transformation,' women can find solace in the knowledge that their midlife journey is not one of isolation, but of empowerment. This period of solitude is an opportunity to forge a new path, to redefine one's identity, and to uncover the hidden strengths within.

As women embrace the complexities of loneliness during menopause, they can draw inspiration from this wisdom. By viewing solitude as a transformative force, they can embark on a journey of self-discovery and growth, emerging with a renewed sense of purpose and resilience.

In conclusion, the interplay between societal changes, personal life events, and biological shifts during menopause creates a unique landscape for loneliness. By understanding and embracing these complexities, women can harness the power of solitude, transforming it into a source of strength and empowerment. As they navigate this chapter of life, they can redefine their identities, build meaningful connections, and embrace the beauty of midlife solitude.

2.3 The Invisible Burden: Understanding the Weight of Loneliness

In the quiet corridors of our minds, loneliness often lurks like an invisible burden. It is a feeling that transcends mere isolation, weaving its tendrils through the fabric of our daily existence. For women in midlife, particularly those navigating the complexities of menopause, loneliness can become a profound and multifaceted challenge. As the body undergoes significant changes, the mind, too, grapples with shifts in identity and purpose.

Mother Teresa once poignantly stated, 'Loneliness and the feeling of being unwanted is the most terrible poverty.' This wisdom echoes with particular resonance for women over 50, who may find themselves questioning their place in a world that often venerates youth and vitality. In this exploration of the psychological underpinnings of loneliness, we uncover not only the science behind this pervasive emotion but also its unique implications for midlife women.

Unravelling the Psychological Web of Loneliness

To truly understand loneliness, we must first dissect its psychological components. Loneliness is not merely the absence of company but rather a subjective experience of disconnection. It is a signal from our brains, alerting us to a disruption in our social bonds. For individuals in midlife, this disruption may stem from various sources: children leaving home, changes in marital status, or the loss of a spouse or close friends. These life events can trigger a re-evaluation of self-worth and purpose, leading to an acute awareness of solitude.

Research in psychology reveals that loneliness is intricately linked to our cognitive and emotional states. It can manifest as a perceived inadequacy or a belief that one is unworthy of love and connection. This perception often fuels a cycle of withdrawal, where the fear of rejection or judgment leads to further isolation. In the context of menopause, these feelings may be compounded by physical symptoms such as mood swings, hot flashes, and fatigue, which can affect social interactions and self-esteem.

The Neurological Underpinnings of Loneliness

Delving deeper, we find that loneliness is not only a psychological phenomenon but also a neurological one. Studies using brain imaging techniques have shown that loneliness activates the same neural pathways associated with physical pain. This suggests that our brains interpret social disconnection as a threat to our well-being, akin to the sensation of physical harm.

For women in midlife, this neurological response can be exacerbated by hormonal changes. The decline in oestrogen levels during menopause can affect neurotransmitters such as serotonin and dopamine, which play a critical role in mood regulation and social behaviour. This hormonal interplay may heighten the experience of loneliness, making it more challenging to seek out or maintain social connections.

The Societal Lens: Ageism and Gender Bias

Beyond the personal and neurological aspects, the societal lens through which loneliness is viewed cannot be ignored. Ageism and gender bias are pervasive forces that often marginalize older women, amplifying feelings of invisibility and irrelevance. In cultures that prioritize youth and beauty, women over 50 may feel pressured to conform to unattainable standards or face the sting of societal neglect.

This marginalization can lead to a diminished sense of belonging, further isolating women during a pivotal stage of life. It is crucial to challenge these biases by fostering environments that celebrate diversity and inclusivity, recognizing the valuable contributions and wisdom of women in midlife.

Harnessing the Power of Solitude

While loneliness is often portrayed as a negative state, it is essential to recognize the potential for growth and transformation within solitude. Solitude, when embraced intentionally, can serve as a fertile ground for self-discovery and personal development. It allows individuals to reconnect with their inner selves, uncovering passions and strengths that may have been overshadowed by the demands of earlier life stages.

For women navigating menopause, solitude can be a time to reflect on their journey, reassess their goals, and redefine their identities. It is an opportunity to cultivate self-compassion and resilience, drawing strength from within rather than external validation. By reframing solitude as a space for empowerment rather than deprivation, women can harness its transformative potential.

Building Bridges: Strategies for Connection

Despite the inherent value of solitude, meaningful connections remain a vital aspect of well-being. For women experiencing loneliness, building and maintaining social ties is crucial. This may involve reevaluating existing relationships, seeking out new friendships, or engaging in community activities that align with personal interests.

Technology can also play a significant role in bridging the gap between solitude and connection. Online platforms and social networks provide opportunities to connect with like-minded individuals, share experiences, and offer support. Virtual communities can serve as a valuable resource for women seeking camaraderie and understanding during the menopause transition.

Conclusion: Embracing the Journey of Midlife Solitude

As we conclude this exploration of loneliness and its psychological dimensions, it is essential to acknowledge the unique challenges and opportunities it presents to women in midlife. By understanding the interplay of psychological, neurological, and societal factors, we can better navigate the complexities of this experience.

Armed with wisdom and strategies for embracing solitude, women can embark on a transformative journey of self-discovery and empowerment. In the words of Mother Teresa, recognizing loneliness as a form of poverty compels us to seek connection, both with ourselves and others, reinforcing the belief that we are never truly alone. By embracing midlife solitude, we open the door to a richer, more fulfilling chapter of life, where the quiet reflections of our inner selves become a source of strength and inspiration.

2.4 Embracing Solitude with Understanding and Action

In exploring the intricate relationship between loneliness and its psychological and physiological impacts, we uncover a poignant truth: loneliness is not merely a state of being alone but a profound experience that can deeply affect our well-being. The studies examined throughout this chapter reveal that prolonged loneliness can lead to significant mental and physical health challenges, underscoring the necessity of addressing this issue with empathy and urgency.

As we analysed how societal shifts and personal life events, particularly menopause, can heighten feelings of isolation, it becomes evident that these transitions require conscious support and understanding. This stage of life, often marked by change and introspection, can be an opportunity to redefine connections and seek new forms of companionship and community.

Mother Teresa's wisdom, 'Loneliness and the feeling of being unwanted is the most terrible poverty,' echoes throughout our discussion, reminding us of the profound emotional and existential impacts of feeling disconnected. Yet, it also serves as a call to action — a reminder that by recognizing and addressing loneliness, we can enrich our lives and those of others.

Key takeaways from this chapter encourage us to cultivate mindfulness in our interactions and to actively seek out and nurture meaningful relationships. Whether through joining community groups, engaging in shared activities, or simply reaching out to friends and family, these actions can alleviate the sense of solitude and foster a supportive network.

For readers navigating midlife solitude, embracing these strategies can transform loneliness from a source of distress into a pathway for growth and renewal. By understanding the science of loneliness, we empower ourselves to address its challenges with compassion and creativity, ultimately enhancing our journey towards fulfilling solitude.

Chapter 2: Reflection Time

- Consider the impact of societal pressures on your personal experiences of loneliness. How have these pressures shaped your emotional health?
- How do you perceive the relationship between loneliness and your physical health? Have you noticed any patterns or changes?
- Reflect on Mother Teresa's words about loneliness. How do they resonate with your personal experiences or observations?

CHAPTER 3

Embracing Solitude: The Path to Self-Discovery

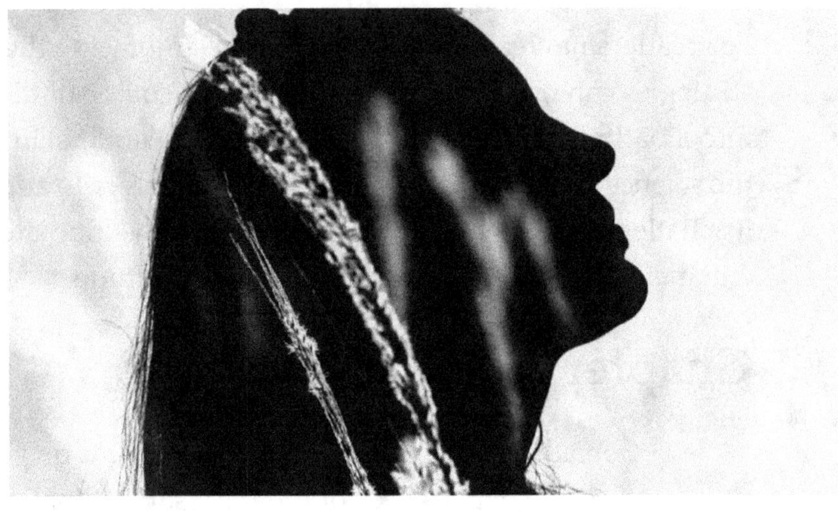

In the tapestry of life, midlife emerges as a profound turning point, a silent transition where solitude often becomes a companion. Yet, within this solitude lies a powerful opportunity for self-discovery—a concept that can transform the perceived loneliness into a reflective sanctuary. This chapter invites you to explore the art of embracing solitude, not as a void, but as a fertile ground for personal growth and deeper self-awareness. As the ancient saying goes, 'Solitude is the soul's holiday, an opportunity to stop doing for others and to surprise and delight ourselves instead.' This wisdom captures the essence of solitude as a time to pause, reflect, and reconnect with the core of our being.

Throughout history, solitude has been revered as a catalyst for transformation, a space where the mind can wander freely and the heart can open to new possibilities. Modern psychological research supports this view, revealing that solitude, when approached mindfully, can lead to enhanced creativity, improved mental health, and a stronger sense of self. For women navigating the changes brought by menopause, such solitude becomes even more significant. It offers a safe haven from the external demands of life and a chance to explore one's evolving identity.

In this chapter, we will delve into strategies that can help transform loneliness into a positive, reflective solitude. We'll explore how mindfulness and meditation serve as powerful tools in fostering a deeper connection with oneself. By practicing mindfulness, you can learn to be present in the moment and embrace your thoughts and emotions without judgment. Meditation, on the other hand, provides a path to inner peace, allowing you to quiet the mind's chatter and tune into your true self.

Consider solitude as a canvas on which to paint the colours of your soul. It is during these quiet moments that you can rediscover passions long forgotten, dreams once shelved, and strengths previously untapped. Solitude encourages introspection, guiding you to question who you are and what you truly desire in this new phase of life. It challenges you to redefine your identity not by societal expectations, but by your own authentic self.

Moreover, embracing solitude offers the chance to cultivate self-compassion and acceptance. It allows you to nurture your inner world, tending to emotional scars and celebrating personal victories. As you journey through this chapter, you will learn how to transform solitude into a nourishing experience, one that fosters resilience and self-awareness.

Remember, solitude is not synonymous with isolation. It is an invitation to embark on a journey of self-discovery, where the only companion you truly need is yourself. By embracing solitude, you can uncover the layers of your being, discovering the strength, wisdom, and creativity that lie within.

As we explore these themes, you'll find practical strategies and insights to help you navigate the path of solitude with grace and confidence. Whether through journaling, meditative practices, or simply taking a quiet walk in nature, the tools you will gain in this chapter are designed to support your journey towards self-discovery and personal growth

In the silence of solitude, you will find your voice; in the stillness, you will find your strength. Embrace this solitude as a precious gift, an opportunity to know yourself more deeply and to emerge with a renewed sense of purpose and clarity. Let this chapter be your guide as you embark on the path to self-discovery, transforming solitude into a celebration of the soul's holiday.

3.1 The Alchemy of Solitude: Transforming Loneliness into Self-Reflection

In the midst of midlife, solitude can often manifest as loneliness, a shadow that creeps into the corners of our lives uninvited. Yet, within this shadow lies an opportunity for profound transformation—a chance to turn the base metal of loneliness into the gold of self-reflection. This chapter explores the alchemy of solitude, offering strategies to metamorphose the initial pangs of loneliness into a rich tapestry of personal insight and growth.

Understanding the Nature of Loneliness

To begin this journey, it's essential to first understand the nature of loneliness. Loneliness is not simply being alone; it is a complex emotional and psychological state that can affect anyone, regardless of their social surroundings. According to recent research, loneliness has been linked to increased stress, decreased immune response, and even a higher risk of mortality. For women navigating menopause, these effects can be particularly pronounced, intertwining with hormonal changes and societal expectations.

The Psychological Perspective

From a psychological standpoint, loneliness during menopause can feel like an identity crisis. The roles and responsibilities that once defined a woman's life may shift, leaving a void that loneliness rushes to fill. This is where the transformation begins: recognizing that loneliness is not a personal failure but a universal human experience that can lead to greater self-awareness and purpose.

The Role of Self-Compassion

The first step in transforming loneliness into self-reflection is cultivating self-compassion. Self-compassion involves treating oneself with the same kindness and understanding that one would offer a friend in need. This practice is particularly vital for women over 50, who may be experiencing changes in their bodies, emotions, and social roles. Embracing these changes with gentleness allows for a deeper exploration of the self.

Practical Steps to Foster Self-Compassion

1. Mindful Acknowledgment: Begin by acknowledging feelings of loneliness without judgment. This can be done through journaling or meditation, allowing the thoughts and emotions to surface without suppression.

2. Affirmative Self-Talk: Replace negative self-talk with affirmations that reinforce self-worth and resilience.

This can be as simple as repeating, "I am worthy of love and connection," each morning.

3. Self-Compassion Exercises: Engage in exercises such as writing a compassionate letter to oneself or practicing loving-kindness meditation, which focuses on sending love to oneself and others.

Reframing Solitude as an Opportunity

Once self-compassion is established, solitude can be reframed as an opportunity rather than a burden. This shift in perspective is crucial for viewing solitude as a fertile ground for self-discovery and personal growth.

Solitude as a Space for Reflection

In solitude, we have the unique opportunity to reflect on our lives without external distractions. This reflection can lead to a clearer understanding of personal values, desires, and goals. For women in midlife, this reflection can be particularly empowering, offering a chance to redefine identity and purpose.

Embracing Creative Outlets

Engaging in creative activities during periods of solitude can be a powerful way to explore the self. Writing, painting, music, or any form of creative expression allows for a deeper connection to inner thoughts and emotions, facilitating personal insight and healing.

Building a Sanctuary of Solitude

Creating a physical and mental sanctuary for solitude is an important strategy in transforming loneliness. This space should be a refuge where one can retreat to engage in reflection and self-care.

Designing a Physical Space

1. Choose a Quiet Corner: Designate a specific area in the home that is reserved for solitude and reflection. This might be a cozy chair by a window, a dedicated meditation room, or a peaceful garden spot.

2. Personalize the Space: Fill this space with items that promote calm and introspection, such as candles, soft lighting, inspiring books, or calming music.

3. Regular Retreats: Schedule regular "retreats" to this sanctuary, treating it as an essential part of the weekly routine.

Mental Sanctuary: Mindfulness Practices

1. Mindful Breathing: Practice mindful breathing exercises to centre the mind and bring awareness to the present moment.

2. Body Scanning: Engage in a body scan meditation to connect with physical sensations and release tension.

3. Gratitude Journaling: Maintain a gratitude journal to focus on positive aspects of life, which can shift perspective from lack to abundance.

The Wisdom of Proverbial Insights

To further inspire the journey from loneliness to reflective solitude, consider the ancient proverb, "In solitude, the mind gains strength and learns to lean upon itself." This wisdom encapsulates the transformative power of solitude, encouraging a deeper reliance on personal insight and strength.

Applying the Proverb to Modern Life

Reflect on how this proverb can apply to your own life. Consider the moments when solitude has led to breakthroughs or quiet realizations that have shifted your perspective. Allow these insights to guide you in embracing solitude as a source of strength and wisdom.

Conclusion: The Path Forward

As we conclude this exploration of transforming loneliness into reflective solitude, remember that this is a deeply personal and ongoing process. It requires patience, self-compassion, and an openness to change. By viewing solitude as an invitation to discover the richness of the inner self, you can transform midlife loneliness into a powerful journey of self-discovery and empowerment.

Embrace solitude not as an absence, but as a presence—a presence of self, of insight, and of potential. In doing so, you will find that the quiet reflections of midlife are not only a path to self-discovery but also a gateway to a more intentional and fulfilling life.

3.2 The Mindful Journey: Unveiling the Self in Silence

In the cacophony of modern life, finding moments of stillness can seem like a daunting task, yet it is within the quietude of these moments that profound self-discovery can occur. The practice of mindfulness and meditation serves as a formidable ally in this journey, offering a sanctuary where the noise of the external world is gently hushed, allowing the whispers of the inner self to be heard.

Setting the Stage: Understanding Mindfulness

Mindfulness is a mental state achieved by focusing one's awareness on the present moment, while calmly acknowledging and accepting one's feelings, thoughts, and bodily sensations. Its roots can be traced back to ancient Buddhist traditions, yet it has found a universal appeal across diverse cultures and spiritual practices due to its simplicity and profound impact on mental well-being. Mindfulness invites individuals to engage fully with life, to observe without judgment, and to cultivate a deep sense of awareness and acceptance.

In the context of midlife solitude, mindfulness becomes an essential tool for introspection. As women navigate the labyrinth of changes brought about by menopause, mindfulness offers a way to anchor oneself amidst the emotional and physical ebbs and flows. It creates a space where women can explore their evolving identities, free from the constraints of past roles and future expectations.

The Science of Mindfulness: A Psychological Perspective

Research has consistently shown that mindfulness practices can significantly reduce symptoms of anxiety, depression, and stress, all of which are heightened during the menopausal transition. A study published in the journal Psychological Science highlighted that mindfulness training enhances meta-awareness and emotion regulation, empowering individuals to better manage mood changes and stress responses. This is particularly pertinent for women over 50, who often experience heightened emotional sensitivity due to hormonal fluctuations during menopause.

Furthermore, mindfulness has been linked to increased activation in the brain's prefrontal cortex, the area associated with higher-order brain functions such as decision-making, personality expression, and moderating social behaviour. This suggests that regular mindfulness practice can enhance cognitive functions, offering women a renewed sense of clarity and focus during this transformative stage of life.

Meditation: The Gateway to Inner Peace

Meditation, a cornerstone of mindfulness practice, provides a structured approach to achieving mental clarity and emotional stability. It is the deliberate act of cultivating stillness, allowing the mind to settle and the spirit to breathe. For women in midlife, meditation offers a retreat from the external pressures and a chance to reconnect with the self.

Subsection: The Art of Meditation - Techniques and Practices

There are various forms of meditation, each offering unique benefits and approaches. Mindfulness meditation, for instance, involves focusing on the breath and observing thoughts as they arise without judgment. This practice encourages a deeper understanding of one's thought patterns, helping to identify and release negative self-talk and limiting beliefs often exacerbated during menopause.

Another popular form is Loving-kindness meditation, which focuses on cultivating compassion towards oneself and others. This practice can be particularly beneficial for women in midlife, as it fosters self-acceptance and reinforces a positive self-image during a time of physical and emotional change.

For those new to meditation, guided meditation sessions — available through numerous apps and online platforms — can provide structured guidance and support. These sessions range from a few minutes to over an hour, allowing individuals to tailor their practice to their comfort and schedule.

Mindfulness in Daily Life: Practical Applications

Incorporating mindfulness into daily life doesn't require hours of practice. Simple techniques can infuse moments of mindfulness into everyday activities, transforming mundane tasks into opportunities for self-connection and reflection.

Mindful Breathing

Mindful breathing is a powerful technique that can be practiced anywhere, at any time. It involves taking slow, deep breaths while focusing on the sensation of the breath entering and leaving the body. This practice not only calms the nervous system but also helps to anchor the mind in the present moment, providing a respite from the worries of the future or regrets of the past.

Mindful Eating

Mindful eating involves paying full attention to the experience of eating, savouring each bite, and recognizing the body's hunger and fullness cues. This practice not only enhances the enjoyment of food but also promotes healthier eating habits, which are crucial for maintaining physical well-being during menopause.

Mindful Walking

Mindful walking is another simple yet effective practice. It involves walking slowly and deliberately, paying attention to the movement of each step and the sensations in the feet and legs. This practice helps to ground the body and mind, promoting a sense of balance and tranquillity.

The Transformative Power of Solitude

The journey of self-discovery through mindfulness and meditation is amplified in the embrace of solitude. The solitude of midlife provides a unique opportunity to turn inward, to listen to the inner voice, and to uncover the layers of the self that have been overshadowed by the demands of external roles and responsibilities.

As the saying goes, 'In solitude, the mind gains strength and learns to lean upon itself.' This wisdom is particularly relevant for women in midlife, as solitude becomes a fertile ground for personal growth and transformation. It is in these moments of quiet reflection that women can redefine their identities, embrace their inherent strengths, and cultivate a renewed sense of purpose.

Embracing the Journey

The path to self-discovery through mindfulness and meditation is a deeply personal journey, one that requires patience, compassion, and an open heart. It is not about changing who you are, but rather about peeling back the layers to reveal the authentic self beneath.

For women navigating the complexities of midlife and menopause, this journey offers a profound opportunity for healing and empowerment. By embracing solitude and cultivating a mindful presence, women can transform this period of transition into a time of renewal and self-discovery.

In conclusion, mindfulness and meditation are not merely practices, but invitations to live more fully, to embrace the present moment, and to celebrate the beauty of the self. As women embark on this journey, they are reminded that they are not alone, but part of a greater tapestry of life, where each thread of experience contributes to the rich and vibrant fabric of existence.

3.3 The Art and Science of Self-Rediscovery

In the journey of life, there comes a profound moment when the clamour of the world fades, leaving behind an oasis of silence—solitude. This silence, often unanticipated, is particularly vivid in midlife, a phase marked by transitions such as menopause, which may amplify feelings of loneliness. Yet, this solitude is not a void to be feared; rather, it is a fertile ground for self-rediscovery, akin to a soul's holiday—a retreat from the incessant demands of life to revel in the surprise and delight of one's own company.

Solitude: The Unexpected Gift

The proverb, 'Solitude is the soul's holiday, an opportunity to stop doing for others and to surprise and delight ourselves instead,' encapsulates the essence of this journey. It suggests a paradigm shift, where solitude is no longer a period of absence but a period of presence — an opportunity to reconnect with oneself. For women experiencing menopause, this phase can be particularly transformative. Menopause, with its myriad of physical and emotional changes, often prompts a re-evaluation of identity and purpose. Yet, it also offers a unique opportunity to explore the depths of the self, free from the roles and responsibilities that have, until now, defined one's existence.

Psychological Insights: Loneliness vs. Solitude

Psychological research distinguishes between loneliness and solitude, emphasizing that while loneliness is a painful awareness of being alone, solitude is a chosen state of being alone. This distinction is crucial for women in midlife, as understanding it can transform their experience from one of isolation to one of empowerment. Studies have shown that embracing solitude can lead to increased self-awareness and personal growth.

In a 2019 study published in the journal Personality and Social Psychology Review, researchers found that solitude can enhance personal well-being, provided it is embraced willingly and seen as an opportunity for self-reflection. The study highlights that intentional solitude allows individuals to process emotions, reflect on life experiences, and develop a deeper understanding of their needs and desires. For women undergoing menopause, this means acknowledging the changes in their bodies and minds and using this period as a platform for rediscovery.

The Role of Mindfulness in Embracing Solitude

Mindfulness, the practice of being present in the moment without judgment, is a powerful tool for those navigating midlife solitude. By cultivating mindfulness, women can learn to appreciate their solitude as a time for self-care and self-discovery. Mindfulness encourages a focus on the present moment, which can alleviate feelings of anxiety and depression often associated with menopause.

A 2020 study in the journal Mindfulness demonstrated that mindfulness practices, such as meditation and mindful breathing, significantly reduce stress and improve emotional regulation. By incorporating mindfulness into their daily routine, women can transform their solitude into a period of introspection and healing. This practice allows them to listen to their inner voice and understand their true self, unencumbered by societal expectations and roles.

Reclaiming Identity through Creative Expression

One of the most profound ways to embrace solitude is through creative expression. Whether it is painting, writing, gardening, or any other form of creative outlet, these activities provide a means to explore and express one's inner world. For women in midlife, engaging in creative pursuits can be particularly liberating, offering a fresh perspective on their identity and purpose.

In a 2018 study published in The Arts in Psychotherapy, researchers found that engaging in creative activities can significantly enhance emotional well-being and reduce symptoms of depression and anxiety. Creative expression allows individuals to process complex emotions, express their unique perspectives, and gain a sense of accomplishment and self-worth.

Building a Sanctuary of Solitude

Creating a physical space dedicated to solitude can also be beneficial. This sanctuary need not be elaborate; it could be a cozy corner of the home, a garden nook, or a quiet space in nature. What matters is that it is a place where one can retreat to reflect, meditate, and engage in self-care.

Designing this sanctuary can be an empowering process in itself. It involves choosing elements that resonate with one's soul—perhaps photographs, books, or artifacts that evoke memories and inspire reflection. This space becomes a tangible reminder of the importance of solitude and the commitment to self-discovery.

Embracing Change: A New Beginning

The path to self-discovery through solitude is not devoid of challenges. It requires courage to face the unknown aspects of oneself and to embrace change. Yet, it is in this very embrace of change that transformation occurs. Research in positive psychology suggests that embracing change with an open mind can lead to greater life satisfaction and resilience.

In a 2022 study published in The Journal of Positive Psychology, researchers found that individuals who viewed life transitions as opportunities for growth reported higher levels of happiness and fulfilment. For women experiencing menopause, this means viewing the changes in their bodies and lives as a new beginning—an opportunity to redefine who they are and what they want from life.

Wisdom from the Ages: Finding Inspiration

Throughout history, many great thinkers and philosophers have extolled the virtues of solitude. The Roman philosopher Seneca once said, 'It is not the man who has too little, but the man who craves more, that is poor.' This wisdom reminds us that true wealth lies in contentment with oneself, and solitude offers the perfect opportunity to find that contentment.

The teachings of Eastern philosophy, too, offer insights. The Taoist concept of 'wu wei,' or effortless action, emphasizes the importance of aligning with the natural flow of life. In solitude, women can practice 'wu wei' by letting go of the need to control and instead embracing the journey of self-discovery with grace and acceptance.

Conclusion: The Journey Within

As women navigate the complex landscape of midlife solitude, they are invited to embark on a journey within—a journey that promises transformation and renewal. By embracing solitude as a soul's holiday, they can discover the hidden treasures within themselves, redefine their identities, and emerge with newfound strength and purpose.

In this chapter, we have explored the multifaceted nature of solitude and its potential to be a catalyst for self-discovery. We have delved into psychological research, mindfulness practices, creative expression, and the creation of a personal sanctuary, all of which serve as tools to navigate this transformative journey.

Ultimately, the path to self-discovery in solitude is deeply personal and unique to each individual. It requires an openness to explore, a willingness to embrace change, and a commitment to honouring one's true self. In doing so, women can find not only solace but also inspiration and empowerment in the beauty of midlife solitude. As they turn the pages of their own lives, they will come to realize that solitude is not a void, but a vibrant tapestry of possibilities waiting to be woven into their story.

3.4 Embracing Solitude: A Journey to Inner Peace and Self-Understanding

In reflecting on solitude as a necessary companion on the journey of self-discovery, we uncover its potential to transform loneliness into a sanctuary of introspection and growth. By embracing solitude, we learn that it is not a state of lack but a presence filled with possibilities. Through mindful practices and meditation, we can cultivate a deeper connection with ourselves, unravelling the layers of our being and gaining clarity on our desires, fears, and aspirations.

Remember, solitude is not merely an absence of company but a presence of self. It is a chance to step away from the incessant demands of the external world and instead, surprise and delight ourselves with our own presence. As you navigate this path, consider solitude as the soul's holiday—a time to cherish and explore your inner landscape without interruption.

Key takeaways include recognizing the power of solitude in enhancing self-awareness and creativity, using mindfulness techniques to anchor yourself in the present moment, and viewing solitary moments as opportunities for personal growth. As actionable advice, schedule regular periods of solitude in your daily routine, even if just for a few minutes, to practice mindfulness and reflection. Allow yourself the grace to be alone with your thoughts, and in doing so, you will find a renewed sense of peace and purpose. Embrace solitude not as an escape, but as an invitation to discover the fullest version of yourself.

Chapter 3: Reflection Time

- How can you transform moments of loneliness into opportunities for self-reflection and personal growth?
- Reflect on a time when mindfulness or meditation helped you connect with yourself on a deeper level.
- What activities or practices make you feel most alive and connected with your true self during solitude?

CHAPTER 4

Redefining Identity: Who Am I Now?

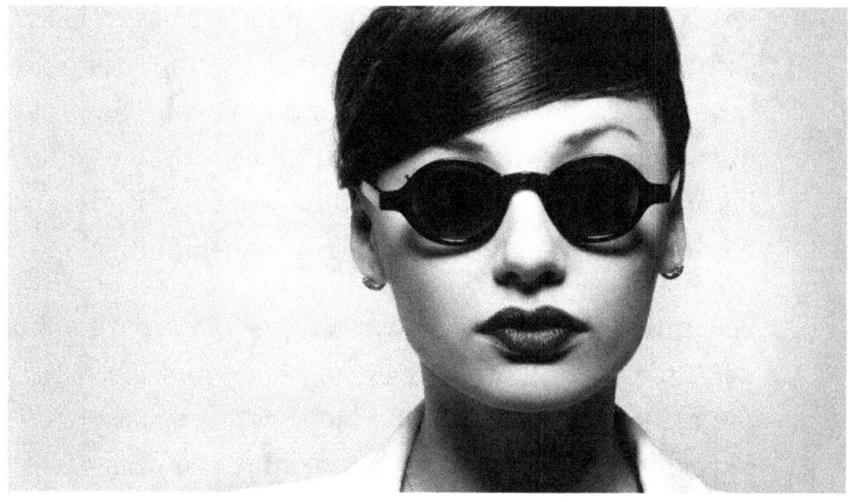

In the tapestry of life, there are moments when the threads unravel, only to be woven anew into a more intricate and meaningful pattern. As women journey through the transformative phase of menopause, they often find themselves standing at a crossroads, questioning their identity and the roles they have long inhabited. This chapter, 'Redefining Identity: Who Am I Now?', invites you to delve into the profound shifts that occur during this pivotal time, exploring the ways in which solitude can be both a companion and a catalyst for self-discovery.

Menopause is frequently accompanied by an emotional and psychological metamorphosis that goes beyond the physical changes. It is a time when the familiar contours of life begin to blur, and the question of identity becomes more pressing. The solitude that often accompanies this life stage can feel daunting, yet within it lies the potential for profound personal growth. Much like the caterpillar that retreats into its cocoon, seemingly at the end of its journey, it is in this seclusion that transformation occurs, giving rise to the butterfly—a symbol of rebirth and renewal. The proverb, 'Just when the caterpillar thought the world was over, it became a butterfly,' serves as a powerful reminder that endings are often the prelude to new beginnings.

Scientific research has shown that the midlife transition, particularly for women over 50, is a period rich with opportunities for redefining identity. According to psychological studies, this stage of life prompts a re-evaluation of personal goals, values, and the very essence of self. As societal expectations shift, there is a unique opportunity to shed past identities that no longer serve you and to cultivate a more authentic self. This process of identity reformation can be daunting, yet it is essential for personal fulfilment and resilience.

This chapter will guide you through this journey of self-reflection and redefinition, offering exercises designed to help you explore your innermost thoughts and aspirations. By engaging in these practices, you will uncover the layers of your being that have been waiting to emerge, much like the butterfly breaking free from its cocoon. You will be encouraged to examine your values and personal goals, allowing you to align them with the person you are becoming. Through this introspective journey, you will find the courage to embrace change and the wisdom to shape your future with intention and clarity.

It is vital to recognize that identity is not a static concept; rather, it is an evolving narrative that we have the power to rewrite. In the quiet moments of solitude, when the noise of the world fades away, you are presented with an opportunity to listen to your inner voice and to honour the truths that resonate most deeply with you. Embracing this solitude as a fertile ground for growth can lead to a renewed sense of purpose and a deeper connection to yourself and the world around you.

As you navigate this chapter, remember that redefining your identity is not about discarding the past, but rather about integrating and celebrating the fullness of your experiences. It is about finding beauty in the intricacies of your journey and using them as stepping stones to the next chapter of your life. In the pages that follow, you will discover the strength that lies within, the courage to embrace new beginnings, and the wisdom to recognize that you are, indeed, becoming the butterfly.

4.1 The Chrysalis of Change: Navigating Identity in Midlife Solitude

The Chrysalis Experience: A Metamorphosis in Motion

Entering midlife is akin to stepping into a chrysalis — a transformative state where one's identity undergoes profound change. For many women, menopause serves as the catalyst for this metamorphosis, prompting introspection and the re-evaluation of long-held beliefs about self and purpose. As hormonal shifts influence mood, energy, and physical health, they also trigger a deeper psychological transformation. Suddenly, the roles that once defined us — mother, partner, professional — begin to fade, making way for new possibilities.

In solitude, women find a space to explore these emerging identities. It's a time to ask, "Who am I now?" and "What do I truly want?" This newfound solitude offers a fertile ground for self-discovery, much like the chrysalis nurturing the caterpillar into a butterfly. Embracing this period of change can lead to an enriched understanding of self, revealing hidden strengths and passions that have been dormant for years.

Hormonal Symphony: The Psychological Impact of Menopause

Menopause is often described as a 'hormonal symphony,' where the ebb and flow of oestrogen and progesterone create a new rhythm for the body and mind. This symphony can feel dissonant at times, leading to confusion and a sense of loss. However, it also heralds an opportunity for psychological growth and identity reformation.

Research indicates that the hormonal changes associated with menopause can influence cognition and emotional regulation. A study published in the Journal of Women's Health found that fluctuations in oestrogen levels can impact mood, memory, and cognitive function. However, these changes also open a doorway for women to reassess their lives and priorities. In solitude, there is an opportunity to listen to this new internal music and let it guide the transformation of identity.

The Wisdom of Solitude: Ancient Teachings for Modern Times

Solitude has been revered throughout history as a crucible for personal growth and enlightenment. The ancient philosopher, Lao Tzu, once said, "Knowing others is intelligence; knowing yourself is true wisdom. Mastering others is strength; mastering yourself is true power." These words resonate deeply with the journey of redefining identity in midlife.

In solitude, women can tap into this ancient wisdom, using the time to master the self. This mastery is not about control but rather about understanding one's true nature and desires. As women navigate the complexities of menopause, solitude becomes a sanctuary — a place where they can reflect on their lives, learn from past experiences, and envision a future that aligns with their authentic selves.

The Role of Reflection: Journaling as a Tool for Transformation

One of the most effective ways to engage with solitude is through journaling. Writing provides a safe space for women to explore their thoughts and feelings, free from judgment or external pressures. It is a tool for reflection, allowing for a deeper understanding of the self and the identity shifts occurring.

Studies have shown that expressive writing can improve mental health and well-being. By documenting experiences and emotions, women can gain clarity and insight into their identity transformation. Journaling can help identify patterns, recognize triggers, and ultimately lead to a more coherent and empowered sense of self.

Releasing the Past: Letting Go to Move Forward

As part of the identity transformation process, it is crucial to release past identities that no longer serve us. This can be a challenging task, as it often involves confronting deeply ingrained beliefs and societal expectations. However, letting go of these outdated roles is essential for embracing a new identity.

Consider the metaphor of a gecko or lizard shedding its skin. Just as the gecko must release its old skin to grow, women must let go of their past identities to evolve. This process requires courage and resilience, but it is a necessary step toward embracing the freedom and possibilities of midlife.

Embracing New Possibilities: Crafting a New Narrative

With the shedding of past identities comes the opportunity to craft a new narrative. This is a time to explore new interests, hobbies, and passions that may have been set aside due to the demands of earlier life stages. Solitude offers the perfect environment to experiment with these new possibilities without fear of judgment.

Women can use this time to discover what truly fulfils them, whether it's pursuing a new career, taking up a creative endeavour, or dedicating time to personal growth and learning. The key is to remain open to change and to embrace the freedom that comes with redefining one's identity.

The Power of Community: Finding Strength in Shared Experiences

While solitude is essential for personal growth, it's important to recognize the value of community and shared experiences. Connecting with other women who are navigating similar transitions can provide support and inspiration. These connections remind women that they are not alone in their journey and that there is strength in solidarity.

Support groups, online forums, and community workshops are excellent resources for women seeking connection during this time. These spaces allow for the sharing of stories, strategies, and encouragement, fostering a sense of belonging and empowerment.

Conclusion: The Beauty of Becoming

The journey of redefining identity in midlife solitude is a deeply personal and transformative experience. It is a time of introspection, growth, and renewal. As women navigate this path, they are reminded of the beauty of becoming—of evolving into a more authentic and fulfilled version of themselves.

In the words of Rainer Maria Rilke, "The only journey is the one within." This journey is not without its challenges, but it is a journey worth undertaking. By embracing solitude, releasing the past, and crafting a new identity, women can emerge from the chrysalis of change empowered, resilient, and ready to embrace the next chapter of life with grace and wisdom.

4.2 The Mirror Within: Exercises for Self-Reflection and Redefinition

Understanding the Essence of Change

As we journey through the profound transition of midlife, the question "Who am I now?" becomes a resonant echo in the chambers of our consciousness. This phase calls for introspection, as it is not just a passage of years but a transformative recalibration of identity that coincides with menopause—a period marked by both physical and emotional shifts. The onset of menopause can amplify feelings of solitude, urging us to redefine our personal goals and values. The ancient proverb, "Change is the only constant," becomes a guiding beacon, reminding us that embracing change is not just necessary but an opportunity for profound personal growth.

The Power of Self-Reflection

Self-reflection is a potent tool in the process of redefining identity. It allows us to pause, observe, and understand the layers of our being. The psychological research on loneliness highlights that solitude, when approached with mindfulness, can be transformative. According to Dr. John Cacioppo, a pioneer in the study of loneliness, the feeling of being alone is a signal that prompts us to reconnect with ourselves and others. Applying this to the menopause niche, women over 50 can harness solitude as a means to explore and redefine their core values and personal goals.

Exercise 1: The Value Inventory

Purpose: To identify and prioritize personal values that align with your current life stage.

Instructions:

1. List Your Values: Begin by writing down all the values that are important to you. These might include family, health, creativity, independence, learning, and spirituality.

2. Rank Your Values: Once you have your list, rank them in order of importance. Consider which values resonate most strongly with the person you are today.

3. Reflect on Changes: Reflect on how these values might have changed over time. What values have risen in importance, and which have diminished? What does this reveal about your growth and evolution?

4. Align Values with Actions: Consider how well your current lifestyle aligns with your prioritized values. Are there areas where you can make adjustments to better reflect your true self?

This exercise serves as a mirror, reflecting the core of who you are now and offering clarity on the path forward.

Exercise 2: Goal Reassessment

Purpose: To redefine personal goals that are meaningful and achievable in the midlife stage.

Instructions:

1. Review Past Goals: Begin by listing goals you set for yourself in the past. Reflect on which ones you have achieved and which remain unmet.

2. Identify New Desires: With your current values in mind, identify new goals that excite and motivate you. These might include learning a new skill, starting a creative project, or engaging more deeply with community activities.

3. SMART Goals: Ensure your goals are Specific, Measurable, Achievable, Relevant, and Time-bound. This framework helps in setting realistic and attainable objectives.

4. Create an Action Plan: Develop a step-by-step plan to achieve these goals, setting milestones and timelines to keep you on track.

Reassessing goals in light of your current values allows a more authentic pursuit of fulfilment and purpose.

Embracing the New You

In redefining your identity, it is vital to embrace the person you are becoming. This acceptance is more than a passive acknowledgment; it is an active celebration of the strengths and wisdom you have gained. Menopause, with its challenges and changes, often brings newfound resilience. As renowned psychologist Carl Jung stated, "I am not what happened to me, I am what I choose to become."

Exercise 3: The Letter to Self

Purpose: To foster self-acceptance and appreciation for the journey you have undertaken.

Instructions

1. Write a Letter: Write a letter to your younger self, acknowledging the experiences, lessons, and growth you have encountered along the way.

2. Express Gratitude: Highlight the qualities and strengths you have developed, expressing gratitude for the resilience that has carried you through challenges.

3. Affirm Your Identity: Affirm the person you are today, acknowledging the transformation you have undergone and the potential that lies ahead.

4. Commit to Self-Compassion: End the letter with a commitment to nurture self-compassion and kindness as you continue your journey.

This exercise is a powerful affirmation of self-worth and a reminder of the incredible journey you have navigated.

Conclusion: The Transformation Furnace

In this chapter, we have explored the profound journey of self-reflection and redefinition during midlife solitude. The exercises presented offer a structured approach to navigating this transformative phase, enabling you to embrace your evolving identity with grace and confidence. As you redefine your values and goals, remember that solitude is indeed the furnace of transformation; it is where you forge the new person you are becoming. By engaging deeply with this process, you can uncover the hidden strengths within, emerging renewed and empowered for the next chapter of your life.

4.3 Emerging from the Chrysalis: Transformative Identity in Midlife

In the tapestry of life, there come moments of profound transformation—times when the familiar threads unravel, leaving us to weave something entirely new. For many women, midlife is such a time, a stage where the question 'Who am I now?' echoes in the corridors of solitude. This chapter explores the metamorphosis that occurs during this pivotal phase, drawing parallels to the timeless wisdom of the proverb, 'Just when the caterpillar thought the world was over, it became a butterfly.' The journey from caterpillar to butterfly is not only a metaphor for personal growth but also a poignant reminder that transformation, though challenging, can lead to unforeseen beauty and strength.

The Chrysalis of Midlife: A Natural Pause

During midlife, women often find themselves in a chrysalis-like state — an introspective pause where external roles and expectations are re-evaluated. As menopause ushers in changes both physical and emotional, it serves as a natural marker for this transition. Research indicates that during this time, levels of oestrogen and other hormones fluctuate, leading to symptoms that can affect mood, cognition, and overall well-being. But beyond the biological changes, there is a deeper, psychological transformation taking place.

The solitude experienced in midlife can be unsettling, yet it is within this quietude that the seeds of transformation are sown. It is a time to reassess personal values, aspirations, and identity. In this stage, the proverbial caterpillar is enveloped in a cocoon — a protective space where it can shed its old self and prepare for rebirth.

Navigating the Psychological Landscape: Loneliness and Self-Reflection

Loneliness, often seen as a companion of solitude, can be a powerful catalyst for self-reflection. Studies have shown that loneliness can trigger introspection, prompting individuals to evaluate their lives and make meaningful changes. For women over 50, this introspection can be an opportunity to redefine their identity beyond societal roles and expectations.

Psychological research suggests that solitude, when embraced, can lead to greater self-awareness and personal growth. Professor John Cacioppo, a pioneer in the field of loneliness studies, highlighted that loneliness can increase self-awareness, forcing individuals to confront their inner thoughts and emotions. This heightened self-awareness can be a double-edged sword—it can lead to self-doubt and anxiety, but it can also foster resilience and clarity.

The Butterfly Effect: Small Changes, Big Transformations

The concept of the butterfly effect—the idea that small changes can lead to significant transformations—is particularly relevant during midlife. As women navigate the emotional and physical shifts of menopause, even minor adjustments in perspective or routine can lead to profound changes in how they view themselves and their place in the world.

For instance, engaging in mindfulness practices, such as meditation or journaling, can help individuals process their emotions and gain clarity. These practices encourage a shift from a negative, self-critical mindset to one of self-compassion and acceptance. By acknowledging their feelings and experiences without judgment, women can begin to see themselves not as victims of circumstance but as active participants in their own transformation.

Harnessing the Power of Narrative: Writing Your Own Story

One powerful tool in the process of redefining identity is narrative therapy—a therapeutic approach that encourages individuals to rewrite their personal stories. By examining the narratives they have internalized about themselves, women can identify and challenge limiting beliefs and assumptions.

Narrative therapy empowers individuals to become the authors of their own lives, allowing them to construct a new identity that aligns with their values and aspirations. This process can be both liberating and empowering, as it enables women to reclaim their agency and envision a future that reflects their true selves.

Building Resilience: Embracing Change with Grace

Resilience is the capacity to adapt to change and recover from adversity. In the context of midlife, building resilience involves embracing change with grace and courage. Research on resilience suggests that individuals who view challenges as opportunities for growth are more likely to thrive in the face of adversity.

For women navigating the challenges of menopause and midlife solitude, cultivating resilience can be a transformative experience. This involves developing coping strategies, such as seeking social support, engaging in self-care practices, and fostering a positive mindset. By focusing on their strengths and capabilities, women can build a solid foundation for resilience and emerge from their chrysalis with renewed confidence.

The Role of Community: Finding Support in Solitude

While solitude is an essential aspect of personal transformation, it does not mean isolation. Connecting with others who are experiencing similar transitions can provide valuable support and encouragement. Sharing experiences, challenges, and insights with a community of like-minded individuals can foster a sense of belonging and purpose.

Support groups, both in-person and online, offer a safe space for women to explore their identity and share their journey. These communities can be a source of inspiration and motivation, reminding women that they are not alone in their transformation.

Conclusion: Embracing the Butterfly Within

As women navigate the complexities of midlife, they are presented with an opportunity to rediscover and redefine their identity. The journey from caterpillar to butterfly is not without its challenges, but it is a journey of immense potential and beauty.

In embracing solitude and the transformative power it holds, women can uncover their true selves and emerge from their chrysalis with newfound strength and clarity. Just as the caterpillar becomes a butterfly, so too can women in midlife experience a rebirth, emerging with wings of resilience, grace, and wisdom. The journey is one of self-discovery, empowerment, and ultimately, the realization that within the chrysalis of solitude lies the potential for limitless transformation.

Emerging from Solitude: Embrace the New You

As we journey through the profound shifts of midlife, particularly during menopause and periods of solitude, we find ourselves standing at a pivotal crossroads of identity. This chapter has delved into the complex layers of identity transformation, guiding you through an introspective exploration of who you truly are. Just as the caterpillar, facing what seemed like the end, emerged as a butterfly, you too have the potential to redefine and embrace a new sense of self.

Through the exercises of self-reflection and redefinition, you have begun to peel back the layers of past identities, revealing the core values and goals that resonate with your current reality. This stage of life is not about losing what once was but about gaining a deeper understanding of who you are beneath the surface changes.

Key takeaways from this chapter include the importance of allowing yourself the grace to evolve and the power of solitude as a space for transformation and renewal. Actionable advice includes regularly setting aside time for introspective practices such as journaling, meditation, or simply sitting in quiet contemplation. Additionally, revisit your goals and values with an open heart, allowing them to align with your current desires and truths.

Remember, the journey of redefining your identity is ongoing and ever-evolving, just as life itself is. Embrace the beauty of this transformation and step forward with confidence, knowing that you are continuously crafting a life that is authentically yours.

Chapter 4: Reflection Time

- How has your identity shifted over time, particularly in the context of menopause and solitude?
- What personal goals and values have become more important to you recently? How do you plan to integrate them into your life?
- Reflect on the proverb about the caterpillar and butterfly. How does this metaphor relate to your personal journey?

CHAPTER 5

Building Resilience: Inner Strength in Solitude

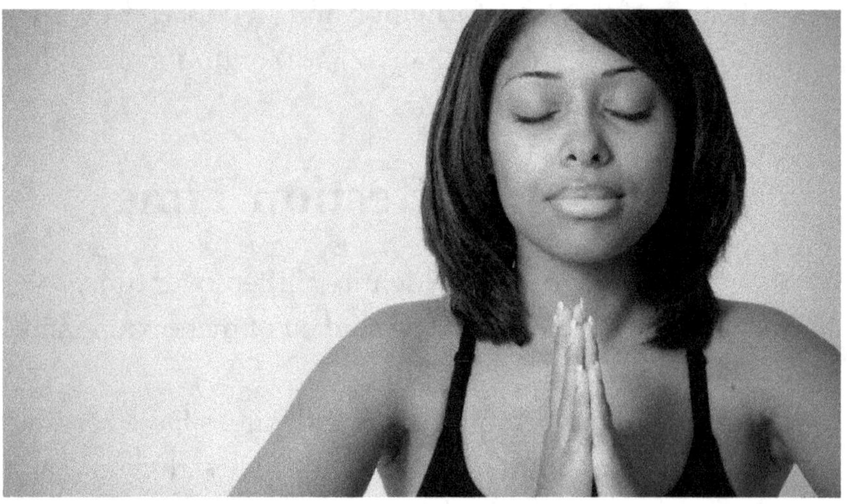

As we journey through the uncharted territories of midlife, it often feels as though we are sailing through tumultuous seas. The storm of solitude can be daunting, yet within its waves lies the opportunity to discover the depth of our resilience—a powerful force that can transform our experience of loneliness into a profound voyage of self-discovery. In this chapter, we delve into the art of building resilience, a vital skill that not only helps us navigate the emotional challenges of solitude but also fortifies us against the wear and tear of life's inevitable hardships.

Resilience is not merely about bouncing back; it is about bending without breaking, adapting with grace, and finding strength in the face of adversity. Imagine the oak and the willow, two trees subjected to the same fierce wind. The oak, strong and unyielding, stands firm but ultimately succumbs to the storm's relentless forces. The willow, on the other hand, bends and sways, yielding to the wind's demands, yet emerges intact. This ancient wisdom — 'The oak fought the wind and was broken, the willow bent when it must and survived' — serves as an eloquent reminder that flexibility and adaptability are paramount in our quest to build inner strength.

In the context of midlife solitude, resilience takes on a unique form. It compels us to confront loneliness not as a burden but as a catalyst for growth and transformation. While the psychological challenges of loneliness can sometimes feel overwhelming, they also present an invitation to cultivate deeper self-awareness and compassion. Research suggests that by understanding the intricate dynamics of loneliness, particularly during menopause, women can develop strategies to mitigate its negative impact. This chapter explores these strategies, providing a roadmap for nurturing a positive mindset and fostering self-compassion — a vital component in fortifying our emotional resilience.

One essential technique in resilience-building is the practice of reframing our experiences. By altering our perspective, we can transform the narrative of loneliness from one of isolation to one of introspection and opportunity. This shift in mindset encourages us to embrace solitude as a sacred space for reflection and personal growth. It is here, in the quiet moments of self-examination, that we begin to recognize our inherent strengths and rediscover the essence of who we are beyond societal roles and expectations.

Another cornerstone of resilience is maintaining a positive outlook, even in the face of adversity. This does not imply ignoring the reality of our challenges but rather choosing to focus on our capacity to overcome them. Cultivating gratitude, finding joy in small victories, and celebrating personal achievements — no matter how minor — are powerful ways to reinforce a positive mindset. Such practices not only bolster our resilience but also enhance our overall well-being, creating a ripple effect that touches every aspect of our lives.

Moreover, nurturing self-compassion is an indispensable element of resilience. It involves treating ourselves with the same kindness and understanding that we would offer a dear friend. Embracing our imperfections and acknowledging our struggles without judgment allows us to build a reservoir of inner strength that sustains us through life's challenges. In doing so, we fortify our emotional resilience, enabling us to face solitude with courage and grace.

In this chapter, we will explore these resilience-building techniques in depth, offering practical strategies to cope with the emotional challenges of loneliness. By embracing the wisdom of flexibility and self-compassion, we can transform midlife solitude into a period of profound growth and empowerment. As we navigate this journey together, let us remember that the storms we face are not meant to break us but to reveal the enduring strength within us.

5.1 The Alchemy of Resilience: Transforming Loneliness into Strength

Resilience is not merely a trait we possess; it is a skill we cultivate, a dynamic capability we can nurture through the trials of solitude. In the realm of midlife, particularly during the transformative period of menopause, resilience becomes an essential ally. It is the backbone that supports us as we navigate the unfamiliar terrain of loneliness, turning what may seem like a barren desert into a fertile ground for personal growth and self-discovery.

Understanding the Nature of Resilience

Resilience, at its core, is often defined as the ability to bounce back from adversity. However, for women over 50, experiencing the seismic shifts of menopause, resilience goes beyond mere recovery. It involves thriving amidst the challenges, embracing solitude not as a void but as a space for reflection and renewal. Psychological research suggests that resilience is not a fixed trait but a set of behaviours, thoughts, and actions that can be learned and developed by anyone.

Consider the proverb, 'A smooth sea never made a skilled sailor.' This wisdom reminds us that it is through facing life's storms that we hone our abilities and fortify our spirits. Similarly, the solitude of midlife can be viewed as an opportunity to build resilience, to become a skilled navigator of our inner landscapes.

The Psychological Underpinnings of Loneliness and Resilience

Recent studies in psychology highlight the paradoxical relationship between loneliness and resilience. Loneliness, often stigmatized, can actually serve as a catalyst for developing resilience. According to research published in the Journal of Personality and Social Psychology, individuals who experience loneliness and actively engage with their feelings tend to develop stronger coping mechanisms over time. This engagement leads to greater self-awareness and emotional intelligence, both critical components of resilience.

For women in menopause, this period of life is marked by profound hormonal changes that can amplify feelings of loneliness and emotional vulnerability. Yet, it is within this crucible that resilience can be forged. The key lies in acknowledging these feelings without judgment and using them as a springboard to explore one's inner world.

Practical Techniques for Building Resilience

1. Mindful Self-Compassion

One of the most effective techniques for building resilience is the practice of mindful self-compassion. This involves treating oneself with the same kindness and understanding that one would offer a dear friend. Kristin Neff, a pioneer in this field, suggests that self-compassion involves three core components: self-kindness, common humanity, and mindfulness.

- Self-Kindness: Instead of criticizing oneself for feeling lonely or inadequate, self-kindness encourages a gentle and supportive internal dialogue.
- Common Humanity: Recognizing that loneliness is a universal human experience helps to reduce feelings of isolation and fosters a sense of connection with others.
- Mindfulness: Being present with one's emotions without over-identifying with them allows for greater clarity and calmness.

2. Cognitive Restructuring

Cognitive restructuring is a technique rooted in cognitive-behavioural therapy (CBT) that involves identifying and challenging negative thought patterns. For women in midlife, cognitive restructuring can help reframe perceptions of loneliness from a negative state to an opportunity for growth.

- Identifying Negative Thoughts: Start by becoming aware of thoughts that contribute to feelings of loneliness, such as 'I am alone because no one cares about me.'
- Challenging These Thoughts: Question the validity of these thoughts by seeking evidence for and against them.
- Adopting a Balanced Perspective: Replace negative thoughts with more balanced and realistic perspectives, such as 'I am alone right now, but this is a chance for self-reflection and growth.'

3. Emotional Resilience Training

Emotional resilience refers to the ability to adapt to emotional challenges and bounce back from setbacks. This can be cultivated through specific practices that enhance emotional regulation and stability.

- Emotion Regulation: Techniques such as deep breathing, meditation, and progressive muscle relaxation can help manage stress and anxiety, promoting emotional balance.
- Positive Visualization: Envisioning positive outcomes and scenarios can shift focus away from loneliness and towards possibilities and potential.
- Gratitude Journaling: Regularly writing down things you are grateful for can shift attention from

what is lacking to what is abundant, fostering a more resilient mindset.

The Role of Social Connections in Resilience

While solitude is a powerful context for building resilience, social connections play a crucial role in this process. Research from the American Psychological Association indicates that social support acts as a buffer against the adverse effects of loneliness, enhancing resilience.

1. Cultivating Meaningful Relationships

In midlife, the nature of social relationships often shifts. Friendships may evolve, and family dynamics can change. Actively seeking and nurturing meaningful connections can provide emotional sustenance and strengthen resilience.

- Join Support Groups: Engaging with support groups, especially those focused on menopause and midlife transitions, can offer a sense of community and shared understanding.
- Rekindle Old Friendships: Revisiting past relationships can bring comfort and continuity, reinforcing a sense of belonging.
- Volunteer: Contributing to community initiatives or volunteering can foster a sense of purpose and connection with others.

2. Integrating Resilience into Daily Life

Building resilience is not an isolated event but a continuous process that weaves into the fabric of everyday life. Here are some strategies to integrate resilience practices into daily routines:

- Daily Reflection: Set aside time each day for reflection, journaling, or meditation. This practice helps consolidate resilience-building efforts and enhances self-awareness.
- Set Realistic Goals: Establishing small, achievable goals fosters a sense of accomplishment and progress, reinforcing resilience.
- Nurture Physical Health: Physical well-being is closely linked to psychological resilience. Regular exercise, a balanced diet, and adequate sleep can all contribute to a resilient mind.

Conclusion: Embracing the Power of Resilience

As women navigate the midlife journey, particularly the challenges of menopause, resilience serves as an invaluable tool. It transforms solitude from a state of absence into a fertile ground for self-discovery and growth. By embracing resilience, women can harness the transformative power of midlife solitude, emerging stronger, wiser, and more connected to their authentic selves. The journey of building resilience is deeply personal and profoundly empowering, offering a profound sense of inner strength that resonates throughout every aspect of life.

5.2 The Resilient Heart: Cultivating Strength Through Solitude

Embracing the Resilient Heart

As we traverse through the stages of life, particularly during the transformative midlife period, the concept of resilience becomes a beacon of hope and strength. Resilience is not merely about bouncing back from adversity but about embracing the quiet power within, cultivating a mindset that allows us to thrive even amidst solitude. This is especially pertinent for women experiencing the profound changes of menopause, a time marked by both physical and emotional shifts.

In the quiet moments of solitude, the heart is given space to breathe, to reflect, and to grow stronger. The resilient heart is not hardened by the trials it endures but is softened and expanded, capable of holding both the joys and sorrows of life with grace. This section explores the profound connection between resilience and solitude, offering insights and strategies to foster inner strength.

Psychological Insights into Resilience and Loneliness

Psychological research has long delved into the intricate relationship between loneliness and resilience. Studies suggest that solitude can serve as a fertile ground for personal growth, provided it is approached with a mindset of openness and self-compassion. According to a study published in the Journal of Personality and Social Psychology, individuals who experience solitude with a sense of purpose and self-reflection often develop greater emotional resilience.

For women navigating menopause, this period of life can feel isolating, yet it also presents a unique opportunity to redefine one's identity and cultivate resilience. Menopause brings about hormonal changes that can affect mood and energy levels, sometimes leading to feelings of loneliness. However, when solitude is embraced as a time for self-discovery rather than isolation, it can become a powerful catalyst for building resilience.

Nurturing a Positive Mindset

A positive mindset is a cornerstone of resilience. It acts as a lens through which we perceive our experiences and challenges. Developing a positive outlook involves consciously choosing to focus on the possibilities and lessons within each moment of solitude. This does not mean ignoring negative emotions but rather acknowledging them while choosing not to be defined by them.

One effective strategy for nurturing a positive mindset is practicing gratitude. Daily reflections on what one is grateful for, even during solitary moments, can shift the focus from what is lacking to what is present and abundant. This practice does not negate the challenges of menopause but rather empowers women to see beyond them, fostering a sense of resilience.

Self-Compassion: The Foundation of Resilience

Self-compassion is perhaps one of the most vital components in building resilience. It involves treating oneself with the same kindness and understanding that one would offer to a dear friend. During the midlife transition, self-compassion becomes an essential tool for navigating the emotional landscape of menopause.

Research by Dr. Kristin Neff, a pioneer in the study of self-compassion, highlights its profound impact on emotional well-being. Self-compassionate individuals tend to experience less anxiety and depression and greater emotional resilience. For women in midlife, practicing self-compassion can help in accepting the physical and emotional changes of menopause with grace and understanding.

The Wisdom of Solitude

"In the solitude of your heart, you will find the strength to face the world," an ancient proverb tells us. Solitude, when embraced with wisdom and openness, becomes a crucible for transformation. It allows for introspection, enabling women to reconnect with their core values and desires, thus fostering resilience.

This wisdom is particularly relevant during menopause, a time that invites profound reflection. The solitude encountered during this life stage can be seen as an invitation to pause, to listen to one's inner voice, and to align with one's true self. In doing so, women can emerge stronger, more resilient, and ready to embrace the next chapter of life with renewed vigour.

Practical Strategies for Building Resilience

Building resilience in solitude requires intentional practice and reflection. Here are some practical strategies:

- Mindful Reflection: Set aside quiet time each day for mindful reflection. Use this time to sit with your thoughts, acknowledging both the positive and negative. Journaling can be a helpful tool to explore your emotions and gain clarity.
- Mind-Body Practices: Engage in mind-body practices such as yoga, tai chi, or meditation. These practices not only enhance physical well-being but also cultivate mental clarity and emotional resilience.
- Creative Expression: Explore creative outlets such as painting, writing, or music. Creative expression allows for the release of emotions and fosters a sense of accomplishment and resilience.
- Connection with Nature: Spend time in nature. Whether it's a walk in the park or tending to a

garden, nature provides a calming and restorative environment that enhances resilience.

- Seek Support: While solitude is valuable, it is equally important to seek support when needed. Connect with friends, support groups, or a therapist who can offer guidance and encouragement.

Redefining Identity Through Resilience

Resilience is not a static trait but a dynamic process of growth and adaptation. As women navigate the changes of menopause, resilience becomes a powerful ally in redefining identity. This period of life offers a unique opportunity to shed old roles and expectations, allowing for a more authentic expression of self.

Embracing resilience involves letting go of perfection and embracing vulnerability. It is about acknowledging the strength that comes from facing challenges with an open heart and mind. By nurturing resilience, women can redefine their identities, creating a life that aligns with their deepest values and aspirations.

Conclusion: The Resilient Journey

The journey through midlife solitude is one of profound transformation and growth. By cultivating resilience, women can navigate the challenges of menopause with grace and strength. This resilience is born not from the absence of struggle but from the courage to face it with compassion and wisdom.

In embracing the resilient heart, women are empowered to redefine their narratives, to find beauty in solitude, and to emerge with a renewed sense of purpose and vitality. As you embark on this journey, remember that resilience is not a destination but a lifelong practice, one that will continue to enrich and empower you in the years to come.

May the wisdom of solitude guide you, and may the strength of your resilient heart lead you to a life of fulfilment and joy.

5.3 The Dance of Resilience: Bending with Grace

In the intricate tapestry of nature, the oak and the willow serve as perennial symbols of resilience and adaptability. While the oak stands tall and robust, it is the willow, with its ability to bend without breaking, that embodies the essence of resilience needed during the midlife journey. This chapter delves into the profound wisdom encapsulated in the saying, "The oak fought the wind and was broken, the willow bent when it must and survived," and applies its lessons to the unique challenges and opportunities faced by women navigating menopause and solitude.

The Nature of Resilience

Resilience is not merely the capacity to endure hardship or recover quickly from setbacks; it is the delicate art of adapting in the face of adversity, much like the willow bending in the wind. Psychological research defines resilience as a dynamic process involving positive adaptation within the context of significant adversity. For women over 50, resilience becomes a crucial ally as they encounter the multifaceted changes of menopause — physical, emotional, and social.

In this stage of life, resilience involves embracing change with grace and finding strength in vulnerability. It demands a shift from a rigid pursuit of stability to a more fluid approach where adaptability and openness to change become vital. By understanding resilience through the lens of nature, women can learn to harness their inner strength in solitude, transforming potential loneliness into a wellspring of personal growth and empowerment.

Embracing Vulnerability

In the quietude of solitude, vulnerability can often feel overwhelming. The changes of menopause bring about shifts that challenge deeply held self-perceptions and societal roles. Yet, it is in acknowledging and embracing vulnerability that true resilience is cultivated. Psychological studies suggest that accepting vulnerability as a natural part of the human experience fosters a deeper connection to oneself and enhances emotional strength.

The willow's flexibility is not a sign of weakness but a testament to its strength. Similarly, embracing vulnerability allows women to navigate the emotional waves of midlife with compassion and self-awareness. By acknowledging fears and uncertainties, they open the door to healing and personal evolution. Vulnerability becomes a bridge to self-discovery, providing the foundation for resilience.

The Role of Self-Compassion

Amidst the solitude of midlife, cultivating self-compassion becomes an essential practice in building resilience. Self-compassion involves treating oneself with the same kindness, understanding, and support one would offer a dear friend. Research by Dr. Kristin Neff highlights that self-compassion fosters emotional resilience and well-being, allowing individuals to better cope with life's challenges.

For women experiencing menopause, self-compassion can be a powerful tool to navigate the physical and emotional changes with grace. By offering themselves understanding and patience, they can alleviate self-criticism and embrace their imperfections. This shift in perspective not only nurtures resilience but also enhances overall mental health, creating a nurturing environment for personal growth.

The Transformative Power of Mindfulness

Mindfulness, the practice of being present in the moment without judgment, serves as a cornerstone in the cultivation of resilience. By anchoring oneself in the present, mindfulness allows women to observe their thoughts and emotions with clarity, reducing the impact of stress and anxiety. This practice enables them to respond to life's challenges with a calm and centred mind.

Research indicates that mindfulness significantly enhances emotional regulation, which is particularly beneficial during the hormonal fluctuations of menopause. By integrating mindfulness into daily routines, women can create a sanctuary of calm amidst the storms of change. This practice fosters resilience by training the mind to remain flexible and adaptive, much like the willow swaying in the breeze.

Building a Supportive Network

While solitude can be a powerful catalyst for self-discovery, it is essential to balance it with meaningful social connections. Building a supportive network of family, friends, or community groups provides an invaluable source of strength and encouragement. Research underscores the significance of social support in enhancing resilience and overall well-being.

For women in midlife, fostering connections with others who share similar experiences can be particularly comforting. These relationships offer a sense of belonging and validation, reminding them that they are not alone in their journey. Through open communication and shared experiences, women can draw strength from one another, reinforcing their resilience in solitude.

Rediscovering Purpose and Passion

The transition into midlife often prompts a re-evaluation of purpose and passion. As roles and responsibilities shift, finding new sources of meaning becomes paramount.

Resilience is fortified by the pursuit of activities and goals that ignite the spirit and provide a sense of fulfilment.

Psychological research supports the idea that engaging in purposeful activities enhances life satisfaction and resilience. Women can explore new hobbies, volunteer opportunities, or creative endeavours that resonate with their evolving identity. By aligning their actions with personal values and passions, they cultivate a sense of purpose that empowers them to navigate solitude with renewed vigour.

Conclusion: The Grace of the Willow

In the journey through midlife solitude, resilience emerges as a dance — a graceful interplay between strength and flexibility. The wisdom of the willow teaches us that true resilience lies not in resisting change but in embracing it with grace and adaptability. As women over 50 navigate the profound transitions of menopause, they can draw inspiration from nature's resilient willow, bending with the winds of change while standing firm in their core essence.

By embracing vulnerability, nurturing self-compassion, practicing mindfulness, building supportive connections, and rediscovering purpose, women can harness their inner strength and transform solitude into an opportunity for profound growth and empowerment. The resilience cultivated in this journey becomes a beacon of hope, guiding them toward the next chapter of life with grace, wisdom, and unwavering strength. Just as the willow survives the storm, women too can thrive in the beauty of midlife solitude, emerging stronger and more resilient than ever before.

Embracing Inner Strength Through Solitude

As we journey through midlife solitude, building resilience emerges as a powerful ally. The techniques discussed in this chapter equip us to navigate the emotional challenges of loneliness, transforming it into an opportunity for growth and self-discovery. By fostering a positive outlook and nurturing self-compassion, we cultivate a nurturing inner environment that supports our well-being.

The wisdom of nature, as encapsulated in the metaphor of the oak and the willow, reminds us of the strength found in adaptability. While the oak stands rigid and breaks under pressure, the willow bends with the wind, embodying resilience through flexibility. In embracing our own 'willow' nature, we learn to flow with life's currents, emerging stronger and more attuned to our true selves.

Key takeaways from this chapter include practical strategies for resilience-building, such as mindfulness practices, journaling, and seeking supportive connections. As you apply these techniques, remember that solitude can be a fertile ground for personal growth. Embrace it as an opportunity to cultivate the inner strength that will guide you through life's challenges with grace and wisdom.

Chapter 5: Reflection Time

- What resilience-building techniques have you found most effective in coping with loneliness?
- How do you cultivate a positive outlook and self-compassion during challenging times?
- Reflect on the proverb about the oak and the willow. How can adaptability and resilience play a role in your life?

CHAPTER 6

Creating Connections: The Importance of Social Ties

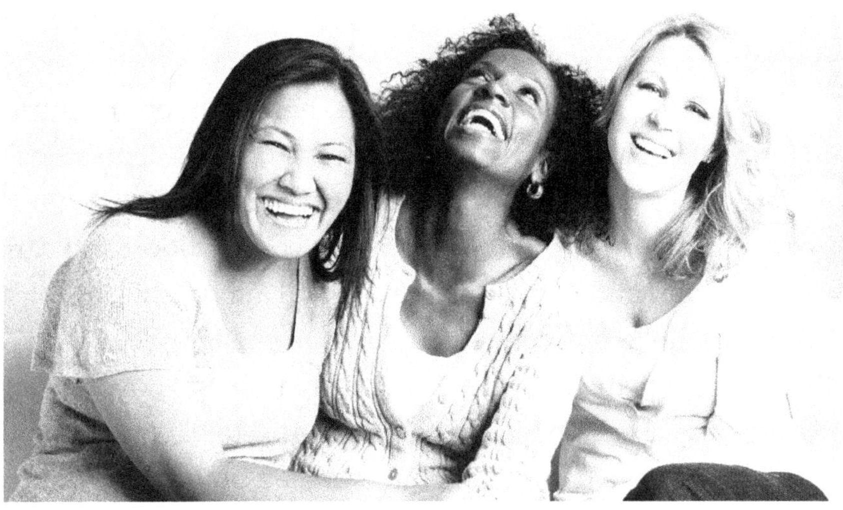

In the tapestry of human experience, few threads are as vital as the connections we forge with others. As we journey through midlife, these connections become not just important but essential, serving as both a balm for the soul and a bridge to a deeper understanding of ourselves. In Chapter 6, 'Creating Connections: The Importance of Social Ties,' we delve into the profound impact that social relationships have on our well-being, particularly in the context of midlife solitude and the transformative journey through menopause.

The proverb, 'A single tree does not make a forest,' aptly encapsulates the essence of our need for community. Just as a forest thrives through the interdependence of its trees, so too do we flourish through the bonds we nurture with others. This chapter explores how, in the midst of solitude, the cultivation of meaningful relationships can mitigate feelings of loneliness and foster a sense of belonging and purpose.

Recent psychological research sheds light on the intricate relationship between loneliness and social connections. Studies have shown that loneliness is not merely a state of mind but a profound psychological condition that can have detrimental effects on both mental and physical health. In midlife, women often face unique challenges as they navigate the changes brought about by menopause, which can exacerbate feelings of isolation. However, understanding the science behind loneliness can empower us to take proactive steps toward building robust social networks.

In this chapter, we will explore practical strategies for creating and maintaining meaningful relationships in midlife. From rekindling old friendships to embracing new social opportunities, these strategies are designed to help you build a supportive community that enhances your journey through solitude. We'll examine the importance of vulnerability and authenticity in forming deep connections, and how these qualities can lead to more fulfilling interactions.

Moreover, we will discuss the role of technology in bridging gaps and fostering connections, particularly for those who might find themselves geographically isolated. While technology cannot replace the warmth of a face-to-face interaction, it offers a valuable platform for maintaining relationships and expanding social circles.

The importance of social ties extends beyond mere companionship; it is a critical component of our overall well-being. Research indicates that individuals with strong social networks tend to experience lower levels of stress, improved cognitive function, and a greater sense of happiness and fulfilment. In essence, our relationships serve as a buffer against the challenges of midlife, providing the support and encouragement needed to navigate this transformative period.

As we embark on this exploration of social connections, let us remember that the journey is as much about giving as it is about receiving. Building meaningful relationships requires effort and intention, a willingness to invest time and energy into cultivating bonds that enrich our lives. Yet, the rewards are immeasurable, offering a sense of connection and community that sustains us through the inevitable ebbs and flows of life.

In the following pages, let us uncover the art of creating connections, discovering how to weave a network of relationships that not only alleviates loneliness but also enhances our journey through midlife solitude. Together, we will embrace the wisdom of the forest, recognizing that while a single tree stands alone, a forest is an interwoven tapestry of strength, resilience, and beauty.

6.1 The Ties That Heal: Social Connections as a Balm for Loneliness

In the labyrinthine journey of midlife, solitude often emerges as a constant, sometimes unwelcome companion. Yet, amid the quietude, social connections can act as a balm, soothing the aching void left by loneliness. This section delves into the profound role that these connections play in mitigating feelings of isolation, particularly for women navigating the transformative phase of menopause. Through the lens of psychological research and age-old wisdom, we explore the necessity of nurturing meaningful relationships to combat loneliness and cultivate a sense of belonging.

Understanding Loneliness in Midlife

Loneliness is not merely a byproduct of being alone; it is a complex emotional state that can permeate one's mental and physical well-being. As women traverse the midlife transition, often marked by the cessation of roles that previously defined them—such as active parenting or career-driven identities—the risk of loneliness surges. Research indicates that this phase can be a unique period of vulnerability; however, it also offers an opportunity for profound personal growth and transformation.

A study published in the journal Menopause found that women experiencing menopause often report heightened feelings of loneliness due to hormonal changes, societal expectations, and shifting family dynamics. These factors can exacerbate the isolation felt during this time, making robust social networks even more critical. By understanding loneliness as a multifaceted experience, we can better appreciate the importance of fostering strong social connections to alleviate its effects.

The Psychological Impact of Social Connections

Social connections are not merely a luxury; they are a fundamental human need. The renowned psychologist Abraham Maslow emphasized this in his hierarchy of needs, illustrating that love and belonging are essential components of psychological wellness. In midlife, the significance of these connections becomes even more pronounced.

Research conducted by the University of Chicago highlights that strong social ties can significantly reduce the risk of loneliness and its associated health issues, such as depression and anxiety. These connections provide emotional support, enhance feelings of security, and contribute to a sense of identity and self-worth. During menopause, when women may feel like they are losing control over their bodies and emotions, the stability offered by social networks can serve as a lifeline.

Building and Sustaining Social Connections

Establishing and maintaining meaningful social connections requires intentional effort and vulnerability. For women in midlife, this can be particularly challenging, as traditional social circles may shrink due to life changes such as retirement, children leaving home, or the death of a partner. However, this period can also be an opportunity to forge new relationships that align with one's evolving interests and values.

Embracing New Communities

One of the most effective ways to build social connections is by engaging with new communities. Whether through joining local clubs, attending workshops, or participating in online forums, these activities offer avenues to meet like-minded individuals. For instance, book clubs, yoga classes, or volunteer groups can provide a sense of camaraderie and shared purpose, which are particularly healing during lonely times.

Nurturing Existing Relationships

While seeking new connections is valuable, nurturing existing relationships is equally important. This involves reaching out to old friends, setting aside time for family, and investing in those relationships that have stood the test of time. Simple acts like a phone call, a handwritten letter, or a shared meal can significantly strengthen bonds and mitigate feelings of loneliness.

The Role of Technology in Fostering Connections

In today's digital age, technology offers unprecedented opportunities to connect with others, transcending geographical boundaries. For women in midlife, who may have been hesitant to embrace these advancements, learning to utilize digital platforms can open doors to new social circles and support networks.

Online Support Communities

Online forums and support groups tailored for women experiencing menopause can provide a platform for sharing experiences, advice, and encouragement. These virtual spaces offer a sense of belonging and understanding, which is crucial for those who may feel isolated in their physical environments.

Social Media and Communication Tools

Social media platforms, such as Facebook and Instagram, can help women stay connected with friends and family across the globe. Additionally, video conferencing tools like Zoom or Skype allow for face-to-face interactions, which are vital for maintaining emotional connections.

Wisdom from the Ages: Proverbs on Connection

Throughout history, cultures across the world have recognized the importance of social ties. The African proverb, "If you want to go quickly, go alone. If you want to go far, go together," encapsulates the essence of this section. It reminds us that while solitude can facilitate quick, introspective journeys, the collective strength of community propels us further along the path of life.

Conclusion: Cultivating a Network of Resilience

As we navigate the often tumultuous waters of midlife, social connections serve as anchors, grounding us in a sense of community and shared humanity. By recognizing the transformative power of these ties, women can embrace the solitude of this life stage not as a source of loneliness but as a canvas for creating meaningful, lasting relationships. In doing so, they cultivate a network of resilience that not only mitigates loneliness but also enriches their lives with joy, purpose, and companionship.

In the next chapter, we will explore how embracing solitude can lead to profound self-discovery, allowing women to redefine their identities and emerge stronger, more fulfilled individuals. As we continue this journey, remember that while solitude is a powerful tool for introspection, it is the connections we foster along the way that truly shape our path to wisdom and fulfilment.

6.2 The Tapestry of Connection: Weaving Bonds in Midlife

In the vibrant tapestry of life, our connections with others form the intricate threads that give it colour and texture. As women navigate the midlife journey, these threads become ever more significant, serving as both anchors and avenues for growth. This section delves into the strategies for building and maintaining meaningful relationships during this transformative phase, with an emphasis on authenticity, vulnerability, and the pursuit of shared experiences.

Embracing Authenticity: The Foundation of True Connection

In the pursuit of meaningful relationships, authenticity is paramount. Midlife often heralds a period of introspection, where the desire to be true to oneself intensifies. This authenticity becomes a magnet for genuine connections. Research in psychology suggests that when individuals present themselves truthfully, they forge stronger and more satisfying relationships. For women in midlife, embracing this authenticity can mean shedding societal expectations and embracing their true selves. This authenticity not only attracts others who resonate with their true nature but also strengthens existing bonds.

The Power of Vulnerability: Building Trust and Intimacy

Vulnerability, often perceived as a weakness, is a profound strength in building deep connections. As Brené Brown, a renowned researcher, highlights, vulnerability is the birthplace of love, belonging, and joy. By allowing themselves to be vulnerable, women open the door to deeper understanding and empathy. In midlife, sharing personal stories, challenges, and triumphs can foster a sense of trust and intimacy. This openness invites others to reciprocate, creating a shared space of mutual support and understanding.

Shared Experiences: The Glue That Binds

Shared experiences serve as the glue that binds relationships. Whether it's a hobby, a shared cause, or simply spending time together, these experiences create lasting memories and strengthen bonds. For women in midlife, engaging in activities that bring joy and fulfilment can be a powerful way to connect with others. This could be as simple as joining a book club, participating in a yoga class, or volunteering for a cause they are passionate about. These shared experiences not only enrich their lives but also provide opportunities to meet like-minded individuals.

Reconnecting with Long-Lost Ties: The Power of Rekindling

As women journey through midlife, there may be an opportunity to reconnect with old friends or family members with whom they have lost touch. Rekindling these relationships can offer a sense of continuity and belonging. It provides a chance to reflect on shared histories and create new memories. In the digital age, reconnecting is easier than ever, with social media platforms serving as a bridge to rediscover past connections. However, it is important to approach these reconnections with openness and an understanding that people evolve over time.

Cultivating New Relationships: Stepping Outside the Comfort Zone

While maintaining existing relationships is important, midlife is also an ideal time to cultivate new ones. This requires stepping outside one's comfort zone and embracing new opportunities to meet people. Whether through community events, workshops, or travel, each encounter is an opportunity to forge new connections. The key is to approach these situations with curiosity and a willingness to engage. By doing so, women can expand their social circles and enrich their lives with diverse perspectives.

The Role of Technology: Bridging Distances

In today's interconnected world, technology plays a pivotal role in maintaining and building relationships. For women in midlife, technology offers tools to stay connected with loved ones, regardless of geographical distances. Video calls, social media, and messaging apps provide platforms to maintain close ties with family and friends. However, it is important to balance digital interactions with face-to-face connections, as physical presence often deepens the emotional bond.

Community Engagement: Finding Belonging in Groups

Engaging with the community can provide a sense of belonging and purpose. Community groups, whether centred around hobbies, support, or advocacy, offer spaces for like-minded individuals to connect. For women in midlife, participating in these groups can be a source of inspiration and support. It allows them to share experiences, learn from others, and contribute to the community. This active participation not only fosters connections but also enhances their sense of self-worth and significance.

Navigating Changes: Adapting Relationships in Midlife

Midlife is a period of significant change, and relationships are no exception. As women evolve, so too do their relationships. It is important to navigate these changes with grace and understanding. This may involve redefining the dynamics of long-standing relationships or gracefully letting go of those that no longer serve their growth. Open communication and empathy are key in adapting relationships to align with their evolving needs and aspirations.

The Balance of Solitude and Connection

While building and maintaining connections is vital, so too is the balance between solitude and social interaction. Solitude offers a space for reflection and self-discovery, which can enhance the quality of relationships. It is in moments of solitude that women can recharge, introspect, and align with their true selves. This balance ensures that when they do connect with others, it is from a place of authenticity and abundance.

A Proverb for Reflection: "A Shared Joy is a Double Joy"

As women embark on the journey of creating connections in midlife, the Swedish proverb, "A shared joy is a double joy," serves as a poignant reminder. By sharing joys, sorrows, and everything in between, relationships are enriched, and life becomes more fulfilling. This wisdom underscores the importance of connections and the profound impact they have on happiness and well-being.

In conclusion, creating connections in midlife is a dynamic and rewarding journey. By embracing authenticity, vulnerability, and shared experiences, women can forge deep and meaningful relationships. Whether nurturing existing ties, rekindling old ones, or cultivating new friendships, these connections enrich the midlife experience, offering support, joy, and a sense of belonging. As women weave their tapestry of connections, they discover that these bonds are not only vital for their well-being but also a testament to the richness of their lives.

6.3 Cultivating Connections: The Forest of Our Lives

In the heart of the African savannah stands the majestic baobab tree, its branches stretching wide and its trunk thick with centuries of growth. Yet, despite its grandeur, the baobab is not an isolated entity; it is part of a vast ecosystem, thriving in concert with the myriad flora and fauna that surround it. This natural symbiosis is wonderfully captured in the African proverb, 'A single tree does not make a forest.' In the context of our lives, particularly in the midlife phase, this adage holds profound truth. We are not solitary entities, but rather, we are interconnected beings whose lives are enriched by the presence of others.

The Essential Nature of Social Ties

Human beings are inherently social creatures. Our need for connection is wired into the very fabric of our being. From our earliest days, we seek the warmth and security of others; it is through these initial interactions that we begin to form our understanding of the world. As we transition into midlife, the nature of our social ties may change, but their importance does not. In fact, research has shown that social connections are a vital aspect of mental and emotional well-being, particularly during the transformative years of menopause.

A study conducted by the University of Chicago found that loneliness can have similar health effects to obesity or smoking, underscoring the critical role that social relationships play in maintaining our health. The menopausal transition can be a tumultuous period marked by physical and emotional changes. It is during this time that the support of a strong social network can provide a sense of stability and reassurance. Friends, family, and community can offer not only companionship but also empathy and understanding, creating a buffer against the feelings of isolation that may arise.

The Psychological Impact of Connection

The psychological benefits of social ties are manifold. They provide a sense of belonging, reduce stress, and enhance our overall life satisfaction. For women navigating menopause, having a network of supportive relationships can be particularly empowering. The psychological research into the benefits of social connections is robust. Studies have shown that people with strong social networks are less likely to experience depression and anxiety. They are also more likely to have higher self-esteem and a greater sense of purpose.

During menopause, women may face a crisis of identity as they come to terms with the physical and emotional changes occurring within their bodies. This is a time when the reassurance and validation from social connections can be invaluable. Whether it is through sharing experiences with other women going through similar changes or receiving support from loved ones, these interactions can help redefine self-perception and bolster confidence.

Building New Connections: A Journey of Discovery

For some, midlife may present a unique opportunity to forge new connections. As children grow up and careers evolve, there may be more time to explore hobbies, volunteer opportunities, or community groups. These activities not only foster new friendships but also create opportunities to engage with people outside of one's usual social circle, broadening perspectives and enriching life experiences.

The process of building new connections can be both exciting and daunting. It requires stepping out of one's comfort zone and being open to new experiences. However, the rewards are often worth the effort. Engaging with diverse groups can lead to newfound passions and interests, providing a sense of purpose and fulfilment. Furthermore, these connections often lead to unexpected opportunities and collaborations, further enhancing the richness of one's life.

Nurturing Existing Relationships

While creating new connections is important, nurturing existing relationships is equally vital. In the hustle and bustle of daily life, it can be easy to take our closest relationships for granted. However, maintaining these bonds requires effort and intentionality. Regular communication, whether through phone calls, emails, or face-to-face meetings, helps keep relationships strong. Sharing experiences, both big and small, deepens the bond and fosters a sense of intimacy and trust.

For women in midlife, nurturing relationships can also involve setting boundaries and managing expectations. As roles and responsibilities shift, it may be necessary to renegotiate the dynamics within relationships. Open and honest communication is key to ensuring that all parties feel valued and understood.

The Role of Technology in Connection

In today's digital age, technology offers new avenues for connection. Social media platforms, video calls, and online communities provide opportunities to connect with others, regardless of geographical distance. For women experiencing menopause, these tools can be particularly beneficial. Online forums and support groups offer a space to share experiences and gain insights from others facing similar challenges.

However, while technology can enhance connectivity, it is important to be mindful of its limitations. Digital interactions, while convenient, should not replace face-to-face interactions. Balancing online and offline connections is crucial to maintaining meaningful relationships.

Embracing Solitude Within Connection

While social ties are essential, it is also important to embrace the solitude that midlife can bring. Solitude does not equate to loneliness; rather, it offers an opportunity for introspection and self-discovery. By balancing social interactions with moments of solitude, women can find harmony and fulfilment in this stage of life.

In solitude, one can reflect on personal growth, set goals, and explore new interests. This time alone can enhance self-awareness and lead to greater emotional resilience. By understanding and embracing one's own needs and desires, it becomes easier to engage authentically with others.

Conclusion: A Network of Support

As women navigate the complexities of midlife and menopause, the importance of social ties cannot be underestimated. These connections provide support, companionship, and a sense of belonging, enriching life in immeasurable ways. By cultivating both new and existing relationships, women can create a vibrant network of support that empowers them to thrive in this transformative stage of life.

In closing, remember the wisdom of the proverb, 'A single tree does not make a forest.' Our lives are intertwined with those of others, and it is through these connections that we find strength, resilience, and joy. By embracing the forest of our lives, we can navigate the journey of midlife with grace and wisdom, finding beauty and fulfilment in the connections we cultivate along the way.

6.4 The Forest of Connection

As we journey through the complex landscape of midlife, it becomes increasingly evident that social connections serve as vital lifelines, effectively warding off the shadow of loneliness that often accompanies this stage of life. In this chapter, we examined the indispensable role these connections play, offering not only companionship but also emotional support, validation, and a sense of belonging.

The proverb, 'A single tree does not make a forest,' encapsulates the essence of our discussions, reminding us that while solitude can be nourishing, it is the network of relationships that enriches our lives, providing the canopy under which we can thrive.

Building and maintaining meaningful relationships requires intentional effort and openness. From rekindling old friendships to stepping outside our comfort zones to forge new bonds, these actions lay the foundation for a robust social network. Additionally, embracing technology as a tool to connect with others, joining community groups, or even volunteering can be effective strategies to cultivate these ties.

The key takeaway from Chapter 6 is that while solitude offers its own wisdom, the warmth and strength derived from social connections are irreplaceable. As you continue in your journey of midlife, prioritize and nurture these relationships. Reach out, share moments, and remember that in the forest of life, interconnectedness is what sustains us. Let this be a call to action: take the initiative to deepen existing relationships and seek new ones, ensuring that your midlife is not just a period of reflection but also one of rich, meaningful connection.

Chapter 6: Reflection Time

- Reflect on the importance of social connections in your life. How do they affect your sense of belonging?
- What steps can you take to build and maintain meaningful relationships in midlife?
- How does the proverb about the single tree and forest inspire you to foster community and connection?

CHAPTER 7

The Power of Purpose: Finding Meaning in Solitude

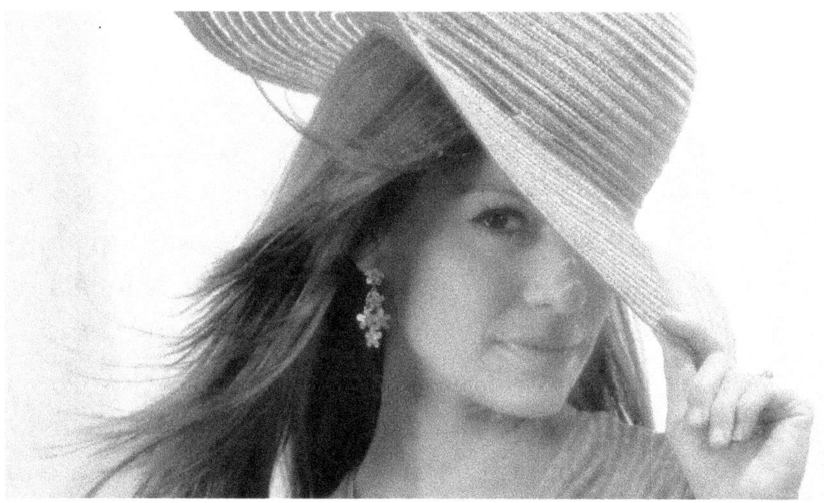

In the quiet embrace of solitude, a seed of transformation lies dormant, waiting to be awakened by the illuminating force of purpose. As we journey through the intricate dance of midlife, the question of purpose becomes a beacon, guiding us through the vast landscapes of our inner selves. It is in this profound solitude that we are gifted the opportunity to reflect deeply, to redefine, and to rediscover our path. The solitude that once felt like a void can become a canvas upon which we paint the vibrant colours of meaning and fulfilment.

The idea that 'The meaning of life is to find your gift. The purpose of life is to give it away,' attributed to Pablo Picasso, encapsulates the essence of what we seek in these midlife years. It is an invitation to look inward, identify our unique gifts, and then extend them outward to enrich the world around us. This quest for purpose is not just a luxury but a necessity, especially during the transformative phases of menopause when the familiar rhythms of life are often disrupted.

Psychological research reveals that the experience of loneliness and solitude is intricately tied to our sense of purpose. A study conducted by psychologist Julianne Holt-Lunstad highlights the detrimental effects of loneliness on both mental and physical health, equating its impact to the risks associated with smoking and obesity. However, these findings also illuminate a path forward: individuals with a strong sense of purpose are less likely to experience the adverse effects of loneliness. Purpose acts as a protective barrier, a guiding star that offers direction and meaning, reducing the perception of isolation.

For women navigating menopause, this period of life can be both a challenge and an opportunity. The shifts in hormonal balance often bring about emotional and physical changes that can feel overwhelming. Yet, it is precisely within this space of change that the possibility for profound personal growth exists. By embracing solitude as a fertile ground for self-discovery, women can redefine their identities and connect with their deepest aspirations.

Engaging in volunteer work, cultivating new hobbies, and embracing lifelong learning are powerful avenues to uncover and nurture one's purpose. Volunteering not only provides a sense of belonging and contribution but also fosters connections with others who share similar values and passions. Hobbies, whether they involve creativity, physical activity, or intellectual pursuit, are gateways to joy and self-expression. They allow us to tap into our inherent talents and interests, offering a sense of achievement and satisfaction.

Furthermore, the pursuit of knowledge and new skills invigorates the mind and injects fresh energy into our lives. Whether it's learning a language, exploring a new field of study, or mastering a new craft, these endeavours expand our horizons and provide a sense of progress and accomplishment.

As we delve deeper into this chapter, we will explore how these pathways not only enhance our sense of purpose but also transform solitude into a period of profound fulfilment and growth. The journey to finding meaning in solitude is deeply personal, yet universally resonant. It invites us to embrace the power of purpose as a transformative force, one that turns the silent echoes of solitude into a symphony of self-discovery and empowerment. Through purpose, we find not only ourselves but also the strength to give of ourselves, enriching the tapestry of life with our unique threads of contribution and connection. Let us embark on this journey together, discovering the beauty and power that lie within the purposeful embrace of solitude.

7.1 Alchemy of Purpose: Transforming Solitude into Fulfilment

Solitude as a Sanctuary for Self-Discovery

In today's fast-paced world, solitude often carries a negative connotation. Yet, when embraced with intention, solitude becomes a sanctuary — a fertile ground for self-discovery and personal growth. For women experiencing menopause, this phase of life can herald a profound transformation, akin to an alchemical process, where the raw materials of one's past experiences are melted down and reshaped into something new and profoundly fulfilling.

Embracing solitude during midlife provides the opportunity to step away from external distractions and societal expectations. It's a time to turn inward, reflecting upon one's life journey, values, and aspirations. This introspection can lead to a deeper understanding of the self, unveiling passions that may have been dormant or unnoticed amidst the hustle and bustle of earlier life stages.

Research in psychology suggests that solitude can enhance creativity and problem-solving abilities. According to a study by psychologist Mihaly Csikszentmihalyi, the state of 'flow,' characterized by complete absorption in an activity, is more easily achieved in solitude. This concept becomes particularly relevant as women in their midlife years seek to redefine their identity and purpose beyond traditional roles. By engaging in activities that foster flow — such as writing, painting, gardening, or even meditative practices — women can tap into a wellspring of creativity and insight, transforming solitude into a deeply rewarding experience.

The Role of Purpose in Enhancing Well-being

Purpose plays a pivotal role in enhancing overall well-being and life satisfaction. It acts as a compass, guiding us through life's challenges and uncertainties. For women navigating the complexities of menopause, cultivating a sense of purpose can be especially empowering. It offers a sense of direction, provides motivation, and fuels resilience in the face of adversity.

Purpose is not a static entity; it evolves with time and experience. In midlife, women often find themselves at a crossroads, questioning previously held beliefs and contemplating new possibilities. This period of transition can be a fertile ground for re-evaluating life goals and pursuing endeavours that align more closely with one's authentic self.

The psychological benefits of having a strong sense of purpose are well-documented. Research by psychologists

Patricia Boyle and colleagues has shown that individuals with a high sense of purpose are less likely to develop Alzheimer's disease and other cognitive impairments. Moreover, a study published in the journal 'Psychological Science' found that individuals with a strong sense of purpose tend to live longer, healthier lives.

Finding Purpose in Passion Projects

One practical avenue for cultivating purpose during midlife is through passion projects—activities or pursuits that ignite enthusiasm and bring joy. These projects can range from starting a small business based on a lifelong hobby to volunteering for a cause that resonates deeply with personal values.

Consider the story of Sarah, a 52-year-old woman who rediscovered her love for pottery during the solitude of her empty nest. What began as a weekend hobby soon blossomed into a thriving small business, where she now teaches pottery classes, sharing her passion with others. For Sarah, this endeavour not only filled her days with creativity and connection but also provided a renewed sense of purpose.

Similarly, volunteering can offer a profound sense of fulfilment and purpose. Whether it's mentoring young women, working with a local charity, or participating in environmental conservation efforts, volunteering allows women to contribute to something greater than themselves. This connection to a larger community can alleviate feelings of isolation and loneliness, transforming solitude into a springboard for meaningful engagement.

The Wisdom of Ancient Proverbs

Throughout history, cultures across the globe have revered the power of solitude as a catalyst for personal growth and transformation. One such piece of wisdom comes from the Taoist philosopher Lao Tzu, who said, 'At the centre of your being, you have the answer; you know who you are, and you know what you want.' This proverb underscores the notion that the answers we seek often lie within us, waiting to be uncovered in the quiet moments of solitude.

This ancient wisdom aligns with modern psychological insights, suggesting that solitude can facilitate self-awareness and clarity of purpose. By embracing solitude as a time for reflection and introspection, women can peel back the layers of societal conditioning and reconnect with their true desires and aspirations.

Navigating the Emotional Terrain of Midlife

The transition into midlife is often accompanied by a complex emotional landscape. Hormonal changes associated with menopause can amplify feelings of irritability, anxiety, and depression. However, by anchoring oneself in a sense of purpose, these emotional waves can be navigated with greater ease and resilience.

Psychologist Viktor Frankl, a Holocaust survivor and author of 'Man's Search for Meaning,' posited that finding meaning in life is essential for emotional well-being. He wrote, 'In some ways, suffering ceases to be suffering at the moment it finds a meaning.' For women in midlife, embracing this perspective can be transformative. By viewing menopause not merely as a biological transition, but as an opportunity for personal growth and self-discovery, the experience becomes less about loss and more about potential.

Practical Steps to Cultivate Purpose

Cultivating a sense of purpose during midlife solitude requires intentionality and self-reflection. Here are some practical steps to help women navigate this journey:

1. Reflect on Past Experiences: Take time to journal about past experiences that brought joy and fulfilment. Consider how these moments can inform current pursuits and passions.

2. Set Intentional Goals: Establish clear, intentional goals that align with personal values and aspirations. These goals should be flexible and adaptable to accommodate the evolving nature of purpose.

3. Engage in Mindful Practices: Mindful practices such as meditation, yoga, or tai chi can enhance self-awareness and clarity of purpose. These practices encourage a deeper connection to the present moment and foster inner peace.

4. Seek Supportive Communities: Connect with like-minded individuals or support groups that share similar interests or life stages. These communities can provide encouragement, inspiration, and a sense of belonging.

5. Embrace Lifelong Learning: Pursue opportunities for learning and growth, whether through formal education, workshops, or self-directed study. Lifelong learning fosters curiosity and keeps the mind engaged.

6. Celebrate Small Victories: Acknowledge and celebrate small achievements along the journey to cultivating purpose. These victories serve as reminders of progress and reinforce the sense of fulfilment.

Conclusion: Embracing the Gift of Solitude

In the tapestry of life, midlife solitude emerges as a unique thread—an opportunity to weave new patterns of purpose and fulfilment. By embracing solitude with open arms, women can embark on a journey of self-discovery, redefining their identity and uncovering the hidden strengths within.

As the ancient proverb aptly reminds us, 'Solitude is the furnace of transformation.' It is within this sacred space that women can find the courage to embrace change, cultivate resilience, and ultimately, transform solitude into a source of profound fulfilment and meaning. In doing so, they not only enrich their own lives but also inspire those around them to embrace the beauty of midlife solitude.

7.2 The Canvas of Solitude: Painting Purpose with New Passions

Midlife is often viewed as a time of reflection, a period when one can look back at the journey thus far and assess the path ahead. It is a phase where the solitude that comes with age can be transformed from a state of loneliness into a powerful canvas upon which new passions and purposes can be painted. The concept of finding meaning through volunteer work, hobbies, and new learning opportunities is particularly compelling for women experiencing menopause. This stage of life, rich with both challenges and opportunities, can be an ideal time to explore new avenues that not only enrich the soul but also provide a renewed sense of purpose.

Volunteer Work: The Joy of Giving

Volunteering offers a unique opportunity to connect with others and contribute to the community, creating a sense of belonging and purpose. According to research published in the Journal of Social Issues, volunteering has been shown to reduce feelings of isolation and improve overall mental health, providing tangible benefits to those who give their time and energy to help others. For women navigating the shifts of menopause, engaging in volunteer work can be particularly beneficial.

The act of helping others can foster a new sense of identity, one that is not solely tied to past roles such as career or family responsibilities. Volunteering can also introduce women to new social networks, offering a diverse array of interactions that enrich their lives. Whether it's mentoring young professionals, participating in community clean-up projects, or offering skills to nonprofit organizations, the opportunities are vast and varied.

A powerful example of this can be seen in the story of Linda, a 52-year-old woman who found herself grappling with loneliness after her children left for college. Feeling adrift, she decided to volunteer at a local animal shelter. The experience not only filled her days with purpose but also introduced her to a community of like-minded individuals who shared her passion for animal welfare. The bonds she formed and the fulfilment she gained from helping animals in need provided Linda with a profound sense of purpose that transformed her midlife solitude into a period of personal growth.

Hobbies: Rediscovering Joy Through Passion

Hobbies are more than just a way to pass the time; they are an avenue for self-expression and creativity. Engaging in activities that ignite passion can serve as a powerful antidote to the solitude experienced during midlife. The psychological benefits of hobbies are well-documented, with studies highlighting their ability to reduce stress, enhance mood, and provide a sense of accomplishment.

For women over 50, rediscovering or developing new hobbies can be a transformative experience. Whether it's painting, gardening, knitting, or writing, hobbies offer a chance to explore new facets of one's identity, free from the pressures of daily life. The process of learning and creating fosters a sense of agency and control, empowering women to embrace their individuality.

Consider the case of Maria, a 55-year-old woman who discovered a passion for painting. Initially taking up the brush as a way to cope with the emotional fluctuations of menopause, she soon found that painting became a meditative practice, a window into her inner world. The colours and strokes allowed her to express emotions that words could not, bringing her a deep sense of peace and satisfaction. Through her art, Maria found a renewed sense of purpose and joy, transforming her solitude into a period of self-discovery and creativity.

New Learning Opportunities: Expanding Horizons

The pursuit of knowledge is a lifelong journey, and midlife offers a unique opportunity to explore new learning avenues. Engaging in educational activities not only stimulates the mind but also provides a sense of accomplishment and purpose. Whether it's enrolling in online courses, attending workshops, or joining book clubs, the options for continued learning are limitless.

For women experiencing menopause, educational pursuits can serve as a powerful tool for personal development. Learning new skills or delving into topics of interest can reignite curiosity and passion, providing a sense of achievement and fulfilment. The cognitive benefits of lifelong learning are also significant, with research indicating that continuous mental stimulation can enhance memory, improve problem-solving skills, and delay cognitive decline.

Take the story of Sarah, a 57-year-old woman who decided to learn a new language. Inspired by her travels, she enrolled in an online language course, dedicating time each day to study and practice. The process of learning not only challenged her mind but also connected her with a global community of learners. The sense of accomplishment she felt with each new word and conversation fuelled her motivation, providing a meaningful purpose that enriched her daily life.

The Transformative Power of Purpose

Finding purpose in solitude is not merely about filling time; it is about engaging in activities that resonate with one's true self, fostering growth and fulfilment. Volunteer work, hobbies, and new learning opportunities offer pathways to discovering and nurturing this purpose. For women over 50, these avenues provide a chance to redefine their identities, embrace their strengths, and cultivate a life rich with meaning and connection.

The proverb "The journey of a thousand miles begins with a single step" serves as a poignant reminder that every new endeavour, no matter how small, can lead to profound transformation. By taking that first step, women can embark on a journey of self-discovery, one that transforms midlife solitude into a period of empowerment and joy.

Conclusion: Embracing the Beauty of Midlife Solitude

As women navigate the complexities of menopause and midlife, finding purpose through volunteer work, hobbies, and new learning opportunities can be a beacon of hope and empowerment. These pursuits offer a chance to connect with others, explore passions, and expand horizons, enriching the tapestry of life with colour and meaning.

By embracing these opportunities, women can transform the quiet reflections of solitude into a powerful catalyst for growth and resilience. In doing so, they not only enrich their own lives but also contribute to the world around them, painting a canvas of purpose and fulfilment that shines brightly in the tapestry of midlife.

7.3 The Symphony of Solitude: Discovering and Sharing Your Unique Gift

In the symphonic orchestra of life, each of us plays our own instrument, contributing to the harmony of the whole. The journey of discovering one's unique gift, especially during midlife, is akin to tuning an instrument to its fullest potential. It is a journey marked by introspection, creativity, and the profound realization that our gifts are not just for ourselves but meant to be shared with the world.

The Search Within: Finding Your Unique Gift

The first step in this journey is to embark on an inward voyage to uncover the essence of who you are. Often, this involves revisiting dreams and passions that may have been set aside in the hustle of earlier years. For women navigating the transformative phase of menopause, this period can offer a unique opportunity to pause and reflect.

Psychological research indicates that midlife is a time when individuals naturally shift from a focus on external achievements to internal fulfilment. This transition is particularly poignant for women, as menopause heralds a new chapter, both biologically and emotionally. It's a time to delve deep into what truly matters to you, what makes your heart sing, and what gifts you possess that can illuminate not just your path but others' as well.

The Gift of Self-Reflection

Self-reflection is a powerful tool in the discovery of your unique gift. Consider setting aside regular time for solitude, where you can engage in activities like journaling, meditation, or simply being in nature. These moments of quiet reflection can help distil the noise of daily life, allowing your true passions and strengths to emerge.

Reflect on questions such as: What activities bring me joy? When do I feel most alive and engaged? What feedback do I consistently receive from others about my strengths? Through these inquiries, you can begin to identify patterns and insights that point to your unique gift.

The Science of Purpose: Aligning Your Gift with Meaning

Research in positive psychology emphasizes the importance of aligning one's gifts with a sense of purpose. Viktor Frankl, a renowned psychologist, asserted that the search for meaning is a fundamental human drive. For women in midlife, this search can take on new dimensions, as personal and professional roles evolve.

A study conducted by the University of Zurich found that individuals who perceive their life as meaningful report higher levels of well-being and satisfaction. This aligns with the idea that discovering and embracing your unique gift can enhance your life experience, providing a sense of fulfilment and direction.

Sharing Your Gift: The Ripple Effect

Once you've identified your unique gift, the next step is to share it with the world. This act of giving not only benefits others but also brings deeper rewards to the giver. The proverb, "The meaning of life is to find your gift. The purpose of life is to give it away," encapsulates this beautifully.

Consider how your gift can be shared in various contexts — be it through volunteering, mentoring, creating art, or initiating community projects. The act of giving transcends the immediate circle and creates ripples that can inspire and uplift others, fostering a sense of connection and community.

The Role of Community in Amplifying Your Gift

Engaging with a community that shares your values and interests can be enriching. It provides a platform to both give and receive support, creating a synergistic environment where gifts can flourish. Whether it's joining a local club, participating in online forums, or attending workshops, these connections can enhance your sense of purpose and belonging.

Embracing Vulnerability: The Courage to Share

Sharing your gift requires vulnerability and courage. It involves stepping out of your comfort zone and embracing the possibility of failure. However, it is through these experiences that growth and transformation occur. Brene Brown, a leading researcher on vulnerability, emphasizes that daring to share our gifts is an act of courage that can lead to profound personal and collective transformation.

The Transformative Power of Purpose in Midlife

The journey of discovering and sharing your unique gift in midlife is not just about personal fulfilment; it is about transformation. It is about stepping into a new phase of life with grace, wisdom, and a renewed sense of purpose. As you embrace this journey, remember that your gift is a beacon—a light that, when shared, can illuminate the path for others.

In the quiet solitude of midlife, may you find the symphony of your soul and the courage to share it with the world, creating a legacy of purpose and meaning that transcends time.

7.4 Embracing Purpose in Solitude

As we journey through the profound landscape of midlife solitude, the power of purpose emerges as a guiding star.

Discovering purpose transforms solitude from a mere state of being alone into a rich, fulfilling experience. By engaging in volunteer work, diving into hobbies, or embracing new learning opportunities, we anchor ourselves to something greater, thereby infusing our solitary moments with meaning and direction. The wisdom that 'The meaning of life is to find your gift. The purpose of life is to give it away,' serves as a beacon, reminding us that in sharing our unique gifts, we unlock the true potential of our solitude.

Key Takeaways:

1. Purpose transforms solitude from isolation into a fulfilling and enriching experience.

2. Volunteer work, hobbies, and learning are effective pathways to discovering and nurturing a sense of purpose.

3. Giving away your discovered gifts not only enriches others but also deepens your own fulfilment.

Actionable Advice:

- Reflect on what brings you joy and consider how you might use that to serve others.
- Dedicate time regularly to activities that align with your sense of purpose, whether it be a new hobby or volunteering.
- Embrace new learning opportunities as a way to continually grow and redefine your purpose.

In solitude, purpose is not merely a destination but a journey that invites us to explore, discover, and ultimately share our gifts with the world.

Chapter 7: Reflection Time

- How does having a sense of purpose transform your experience of solitude into fulfilment?
- What activities or interests ignite your sense of purpose, and how can you incorporate them into your daily life?
- Reflect on the wisdom about finding and giving your gift. What unique gifts do you have to offer the world?

CHAPTER 8

Navigating Emotional Waves: Managing Mood Changes

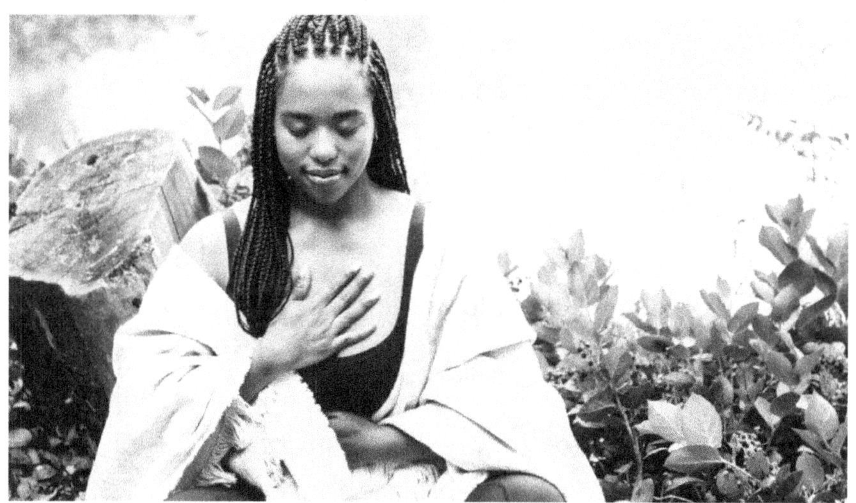

As the sun rises over the horizon, painting the sky with hues of hope and promise, so too do the emotional currents of midlife begin to shift and change, bringing with them a symphony of experiences that are both challenging and transformative. Chapter 8, 'Navigating Emotional Waves: Managing Mood Changes,' invites you to embark on a journey through the intricate emotional landscape of menopause, a time often characterized by its unpredictable shifts in mood and temperament. This chapter serves as a compass, guiding you through the turbulent seas of emotional change, armed with the wisdom and strategies necessary to not only weather the storm but to emerge from it more resilient and self-assured.

The proverb, 'Smooth seas do not make skilful sailors,' elegantly encapsulates the essence of this journey. It reminds us that it is through navigating life's challenges, rather than avoiding them, that we cultivate strength, wisdom, and resilience. The emotional fluctuations that accompany menopause are akin to waves crashing against the shore, sometimes gentle and rhythmic, other times powerful and overwhelming. They test our mettle and force us to confront the depths of our own psychological resilience.

In the realm of psychological research, the link between mood changes and loneliness during menopause is a well-documented phenomenon. Studies indicate that hormonal fluctuations can lead to mood swings, irritability, and even bouts of depression, which, if left unaddressed, may contribute to feelings of isolation and loneliness. This chapter delves into the science underpinning these changes, offering a nuanced understanding of the biological and psychological factors at play. By unravelling the complexities of mood fluctuations, we can begin to demystify the emotions that often feel beyond our control, empowering ourselves with the knowledge needed to manage these changes effectively.

Yet, understanding is only the beginning. Armed with insights from psychological research, this chapter offers practical strategies for emotional regulation and stress management. You will discover techniques rooted in mindfulness, cognitive-behavioural approaches, and holistic practices that foster emotional balance and resilience. These strategies are designed to help you ride the emotional waves with grace, allowing you to find moments of calm amidst the storm.

Moreover, 'Navigating Emotional Waves' emphasizes the importance of viewing these mood changes not as adversaries, but as opportunities for growth and self-reflection. By embracing these emotional shifts, we can uncover deeper insights into our personal needs, desires, and aspirations. This perspective shift transforms what may initially feel like chaos into a fertile ground for self-discovery and transformation, aligning with the overarching theme of solitude as a furnace of transformation

As you delve into this chapter, let it be a reminder that you are not alone in this journey. Countless others have traversed these same waters, emerging stronger and more self-aware on the other side. With the guidance and strategies laid out before you, you too can become a skilful sailor, navigating the emotional waves of menopause with confidence, resilience, and a renewed sense of purpose. Together, let us embrace the beauty of this transformative journey, finding strength in solitude and wisdom in the waves.

8.1 The Emotional Pendulum: Understanding Mood Fluctuations in Menopause

Unravelling the Emotional Labyrinth

As women navigate the complex journey of menopause, they often encounter a myriad of emotional challenges that can be as bewildering as they are intense. These mood fluctuations, akin to riding an emotional pendulum, are not mere figments of imagination but are deeply rooted in the physiological changes occurring within the body. Understanding this emotional labyrinth is the first step toward managing its impact on loneliness and embracing the solitude that often accompanies this life stage.

During menopause, the body undergoes significant hormonal shifts, primarily characterized by declining levels of oestrogen and progesterone. These hormones, which have been regulating various bodily functions for decades, are intricately linked to the brain's chemistry and mood regulation. The sudden decrease in oestrogen levels can lead to increased production of stress hormones like cortisol, which can exacerbate feelings of anxiety and depression. Moreover, oestrogen is known to influence serotonin, a neurotransmitter that plays a crucial role in mood regulation. As serotonin levels fluctuate, women may experience heightened emotional sensitivity, mood swings, and irritability.

The psychological impact of these hormonal changes can be profound, often leading to a sense of loneliness and isolation. Many women find themselves grappling with emotions they struggle to articulate or understand, feeling disconnected from their previous selves and the world around them. This emotional upheaval can be particularly challenging for those who have not previously experienced significant mood disorders, leaving them feeling unprepared and vulnerable.

The Cycle of Loneliness and Emotional Vulnerability

Loneliness during menopause is not merely a byproduct of physical changes; it is a complex interplay of emotional, social, and psychological factors. The emotional vulnerability induced by hormonal fluctuations can create a fertile ground for loneliness to thrive. As women encounter mood swings, they may withdraw from social interactions, fearing judgment or misunderstanding from others. This withdrawal can lead to a self-perpetuating cycle of loneliness, where isolation breeds further emotional distress.

In the context of menopause, loneliness is often exacerbated by societal attitudes and misconceptions. Many women feel the pressure to maintain a facade of strength and composure, despite the emotional turmoil beneath the surface. The stigma surrounding menopause can lead to feelings of shame and inadequacy, further isolating women from seeking the support they need. This societal silence around menopause can reinforce the notion that these experiences are to be borne in solitude, leaving women feeling disconnected from their communities and support networks.

Harnessing Solitude as a Catalyst for Transformation

While the emotional waves of menopause can be overwhelming, solitude can serve as a powerful catalyst for transformation and self-discovery. In the silence of solitude, women have the opportunity to reflect on their emotions and gain a deeper understanding of their inner selves. This period of introspection can be a time of profound growth, allowing women to redefine their identities and embrace the changes that come with midlife.

Solitude offers a space for women to explore their emotions without judgment, providing a sanctuary for healing and renewal. By embracing solitude, women can cultivate a sense of inner peace and resilience, transforming loneliness into a source of strength. It is in these moments of quiet reflection that women can reconnect with their true selves, shedding the societal expectations and pressures that have burdened them for so long.

Practical Strategies for Navigating Mood Fluctuations

To effectively manage mood fluctuations and their impact on loneliness, it is essential to adopt practical strategies that promote emotional well-being and resilience. One such strategy is mindfulness meditation, which encourages individuals to focus on the present moment and cultivate a non-judgmental awareness of their thoughts and feelings. Mindfulness has been shown to reduce stress and improve emotional regulation, making it an invaluable tool for navigating the emotional waves of menopause.

Additionally, engaging in regular physical activity can have a positive impact on mood and emotional health. Exercise has been shown to increase the production of endorphins, often referred to as "feel-good" hormones, which can alleviate symptoms of anxiety and depression. Incorporating activities such as yoga, walking, or swimming into daily routines can provide a natural and effective means of managing mood fluctuations.

Building a robust support network is another crucial element in combating loneliness and emotional distress during menopause. Reaching out to friends, family, or support groups can provide a sense of connection and belonging, alleviating feelings of isolation. Sharing experiences and challenges with others who understand can foster a sense of solidarity and empowerment, reducing the stigma surrounding menopause and its emotional impact.

Embracing the Wisdom of Ancient Proverbs

In moments of solitude and reflection, it can be helpful to draw inspiration from ancient proverbs and wisdom that have withstood the test of time. One such proverb, "This too shall pass," reminds us of the transient nature of life's challenges and the resilience of the human spirit. By embracing this timeless wisdom, women can find comfort and strength in the knowledge that the emotional waves of menopause, though daunting, are not permanent.

Another empowering piece of wisdom comes from the Daoist philosophy, which teaches that "Stillness reveals the secrets of the universe." This proverb encourages individuals to embrace moments of stillness and solitude as opportunities for profound growth and self-discovery. By cultivating an attitude of acceptance and patience, women can navigate the emotional waves of menopause with grace and wisdom, transforming solitude into a source of empowerment and renewal.

Conclusion: A New Dawn Awaits

As women journey through the emotional landscape of menopause, they are invited to embrace solitude as a powerful ally in their quest for self-discovery and transformation. By understanding the physiological and psychological underpinnings of mood fluctuations, women can develop strategies to manage their emotional well-being and combat loneliness. Through mindfulness, physical activity, and the support of a nurturing community, women can cultivate resilience and strength, redefining their identities and embracing the beauty of midlife solitude.

In the quiet moments of reflection, women can find solace and empowerment, transforming the emotional waves of menopause into a symphony of growth and renewal. By embracing the wisdom of ancient proverbs and the transformative power of solitude, women can navigate this life stage with grace and wisdom, ready to embrace the next chapter of their lives with open hearts and minds. The journey of menopause, though challenging, is also a time of profound opportunity, inviting women to rediscover their true selves and harness the strength within. A new dawn awaits, and with it, the promise of a life enriched by the beauty of solitude and the wisdom of experience.

8.2 Emotional Equilibrium: Riding the Waves of Change

As we journey through midlife, the emotional landscape can feel like a tumultuous sea, with waves of change that threaten to pull us under. However, by cultivating emotional equilibrium, we can learn to ride these waves with grace and resilience. This section delves into the art of emotional regulation and stress management, offering practical strategies to help you navigate the inevitable mood changes that accompany menopause.

Understanding Emotional Waves

In the midst of menopause, emotional fluctuations are not just common—they are expected. The hormonal changes that occur during this stage of life can lead to mood swings, anxiety, and even depression. These emotional waves are akin to the phases of the moon—predictable yet powerful, affecting the tides of our inner world.

Psychological research suggests that understanding the biological and emotional underpinnings of these changes is the first step toward managing them. According to a study published in the Journal of Women's Health, fluctuations in oestrogen and progesterone levels directly impact neurotransmitters such as serotonin, which plays a crucial role in mood regulation. By gaining insight into this connection, women can begin to dissociate their identity from their fluctuating emotions, recognizing them as a natural part of the menopause journey.

The Art of Emotional Regulation

Emotional regulation is the ability to respond to experiences with a range of emotions in a manner that is socially tolerable and flexible enough to permit spontaneous or delayed reactions. It involves managing your emotional reactions to achieve a balance that allows for both personal and relationship growth.

One effective technique for emotional regulation is mindfulness. Mindfulness encourages us to focus on the present moment, acknowledging our thoughts and feelings without judgment. This practice can be particularly helpful for women experiencing menopause, as it fosters a compassionate acceptance of emotional states. A study conducted by Brown and Ryan (2003) suggests that individuals who practice mindfulness demonstrate greater emotional stability and resilience.

Mindfulness in Practice

To incorporate mindfulness into your daily routine, consider the following exercises:

1. Mindful Breathing: Dedicate a few minutes each day to focus on your breath. Inhale deeply, hold, and exhale slowly. This simple practice can help ground you during emotional upheavals.

2. Body Scan Meditation: Lie down comfortably and bring attention to each part of your body, noticing any tension or discomfort. This exercise promotes relaxation and body awareness, helping to release pent-up emotions.

3. Mindful Journaling: Spend time each day writing about your thoughts and feelings. This practice not only aids in emotional release but also provides clarity and insight into recurring emotional patterns.

Stress Management Strategies

Stress is a formidable companion of emotional waves, often exacerbating mood changes during menopause. Effective stress management is crucial for maintaining emotional equilibrium. Here are some strategies that can help:

1. Physical Activity: Engaging in regular physical activity can significantly reduce stress levels. Exercise stimulates the production of endorphins, which are natural mood lifters. Whether it's a brisk walk, yoga, or dancing, find an activity you enjoy and make it a part of your routine.

2. Healthy Nutrition: A balanced diet rich in whole foods can have a profound impact on emotional well-being. Foods high in omega-3 fatty acids, such as salmon and walnuts, are known to support brain health and enhance mood.

3. Social Support: Building a network of supportive friends and family members can provide a buffer against stress. Sharing your experiences and feelings with others who understand can be incredibly therapeutic.

Harnessing the Power of Proactivity

Proactivity is the ability to anticipate and prepare for emotional waves, rather than merely reacting to them. By developing a proactive mindset, women can feel more in control of their emotional landscape.

1. Set Realistic Expectations: Acknowledge that mood changes are a natural part of menopause. By setting

realistic expectations for yourself, you can avoid the guilt or frustration that often accompanies emotional fluctuations.

2. Create a Safe Space: Designate a physical or mental space where you can retreat when emotions become overwhelming. This could be a cozy corner in your home, a favourite park, or a mental visualization of a serene place.

3. Practice Gratitude: Cultivating gratitude can shift your focus from what is lacking to what is abundant in your life. This positive shift in perspective can help mitigate the impact of negative emotions.

Finding Wisdom in Ancient Proverbs

As you navigate the emotional waves of menopause, consider the wisdom encapsulated in the ancient proverb: "This too shall pass." This simple yet profound saying serves as a reminder that emotions are transient, and even the most intense feelings will eventually subside. Embracing this wisdom can provide solace and perspective during challenging times.

Building Emotional Resilience

Emotional resilience is the ability to bounce back from adversity and adapt to change. During menopause, building resilience is essential for maintaining emotional well-being. Here are some ways to cultivate resilience:

1. Embrace Change: Accept that change is an inevitable part of life. By viewing change as an opportunity for growth rather than a threat, you can develop a more resilient mindset.

2. Develop Problem-Solving Skills: Strengthening your problem-solving abilities can enhance resilience by empowering you to tackle challenges effectively.

3. Seek Professional Support: If you find yourself overwhelmed by emotional changes, don't hesitate to seek support from a mental health professional. Therapy can provide valuable tools and insights for managing emotions.

The Journey Toward Emotional Equilibrium

Navigating the emotional waves of menopause is a deeply personal journey. By understanding the biological and psychological roots of these changes, practicing mindfulness, managing stress, and building resilience, women can find emotional equilibrium. As you embrace this phase of life, remember that you are not alone — countless women have walked this path before you, emerging stronger and more self-aware.

In closing, the journey to emotional equilibrium is not about achieving a state of constant calm but rather learning to ride the waves with grace and acceptance. This journey is one of growth, self-discovery, and, ultimately, transformation. As you continue to navigate the emotional seas of midlife, may you find strength in your solitude and courage in your vulnerability. Embrace the waves, for they are the very currents that will carry you toward a deeper understanding of yourself and your place in the world.

8.3 Riding the Emotional Tides: Understanding and Embracing Mood Shifts

The Nature of Emotional Waves: Embracing the Flow

In the midst of midlife, a time often marked by significant transitions and transformations, the emotional landscape can appear like the ever-changing sea. The proverb 'Smooth seas do not make skilful sailors' perfectly encapsulates the essence of navigating mood changes during this phase. Menopause, a significant milestone for women typically occurring in their 50s or older, brings with it a plethora of emotional shifts that might feel overwhelming. However, just as a sailor learns to read the winds and waves, women can learn to navigate their emotional tides, gaining resilience and wisdom in the process.

Understanding the Emotional Shifts

Hormonal changes during menopause are akin to the shifting currents of the ocean. Oestrogen and progesterone, hormones that have been stable for many years, begin to fluctuate, leading to erratic emotional states. These fluctuations can manifest as mood swings, anxiety, irritability, and even depression. Acknowledging these changes as a natural part of the midlife journey is crucial. By understanding the science behind these emotional waves, women can approach them with a sense of curiosity rather than fear.

Psychological research highlights that these mood changes are not solely tied to hormonal shifts but are also influenced by various psychosocial factors. The transition into midlife often coincides with other life changes such as children leaving home, career transitions, or the care of aging parents. These factors can exacerbate feelings of loneliness or loss of purpose. Recognizing the interconnectedness of these influences allows for a more holistic approach to managing emotional health.

The Role of Loneliness in Emotional Turbulence

Loneliness is often described as a silent companion during the midlife transition. Research suggests that loneliness can amplify mood disturbances, creating a feedback loop that intensifies emotional distress. The lack of social support or meaningful connections during this time can lead to feelings of isolation, further complicating the emotional landscape.

A study published in the 'Journal of Affective Disorders' found that loneliness is a significant predictor of depression and anxiety in midlife women. The psychological impact of feeling disconnected from others can be profound, leading to a decrease in overall well-being. However, by understanding loneliness as a modifiable factor, women can take proactive steps to mitigate its effects.

Strategies for Navigating Mood Changes

Embrace the Emotional Experience

One of the first steps in managing mood changes is to embrace the emotional experience rather than resist it. Accepting emotions as they arise allows for a more authentic engagement with oneself. This acceptance does not mean resigning to negative feelings but rather acknowledging them as a natural part of the human experience. Mindfulness practices, such as meditation or deep-breathing exercises, can be invaluable tools in fostering this acceptance.

Cultivate Resilience Through Self-Compassion

Self-compassion, the practice of treating oneself with kindness and understanding, is a powerful antidote to the harsh self-criticism that often accompanies emotional turbulence. Research by Dr. Kristin Neff highlights that self-compassion can significantly reduce anxiety and depression, fostering a sense of resilience. By practicing self-compassion, women can navigate their emotional waves with grace, recognizing that they are not alone in their struggles.

Reframe Loneliness as Solitude

Reframing loneliness as solitude can transform the emotional experience. Solitude offers a unique opportunity for introspection and self-discovery. By viewing time alone as a chance to reconnect with oneself, women can shift their perspective from one of deprivation to one of enrichment. This reframing can lead to a deeper understanding of personal values and desires, ultimately enhancing emotional fulfilment.

Building a Supportive Environment

Strengthening Social Connections

While embracing solitude is beneficial, it is equally important to cultivate meaningful social connections. The proverb 'Smooth seas do not make skilful sailors' reminds us that challenges are opportunities for growth. Building a supportive network of friends, family, or community can provide the emotional buoyancy needed to navigate turbulent times. Engaging in social activities or joining support groups specifically for midlife women can foster a sense of belonging and reduce feelings of isolation.

Seek Professional Support

For some, professional support may be necessary to effectively manage mood changes. Therapists or counsellors can provide invaluable guidance in navigating the emotional complexities of midlife. Cognitive-behavioural therapy (CBT), for example, has been shown to be particularly effective in treating menopause-related mood disturbances. By seeking professional help, women can gain personalized strategies to cope with their unique challenges.

Embracing the Journey: Wisdom in Every Wave

Navigating the emotional waves of midlife is not about seeking calm seas at all times but rather about learning how to ride the waves with skill and confidence. Each emotional experience, whether tumultuous or serene, offers a unique opportunity for growth and self-discovery. By embracing the full spectrum of emotions, women can emerge from this journey with a deeper understanding of themselves and a renewed sense of purpose.

As the proverb suggests, the skilful sailor is not made in calm waters but through the trials faced in turbulent seas. So too are women of midlife shaped by their emotional experiences. By employing strategies to manage mood changes and reframing their perspective, they can navigate this transformative period with grace, emerging stronger and more resilient than before.

8.4 Embracing the Waves: Mastering Emotional Shifts

As we draw the curtains on this chapter, it's essential to recognize that navigating the emotional waves of midlife, particularly those associated with menopause, is akin to sailing through turbulent seas. These fluctuations can amplify feelings of loneliness, yet they also present an opportunity for profound personal growth. Remember, 'Smooth seas do not make skilful sailors.' Embracing the challenges of mood changes with grace and resilience allows for the cultivation of emotional intelligence and strength.

Key strategies for emotional regulation and stress management include mindfulness practices, such as meditation and deep-breathing exercises, which can anchor you during emotional storms. Engaging in regular physical activity and maintaining a balanced diet are crucial in stabilizing mood and enhancing overall well-being. Additionally, fostering a supportive social network can mitigate feelings of isolation, providing a lifeline in moments of solitude.

In conclusion, while the emotional tides of this life stage may seem daunting, they offer a chance to develop resilience and adaptability. By implementing these strategies, you can transform midlife solitude into a period of reflection and growth, ultimately navigating these emotional waves with skill and confidence. Remember, each wave you face is an opportunity to refine your emotional seafaring skills, leading to a more profound understanding of yourself and the world around you.

Chapter 8: Reflection Time

- How do mood fluctuations impact your experience of loneliness, and what strategies help you manage them?
- Reflect on a time when you navigated emotional challenges successfully. What did you learn from that experience?
- How does the proverb about skilful sailors resonate with your journey through emotional ups and downs?

CHAPTER 9

BODY AND MIND: EMBRACING HOLISTIC HEALTH

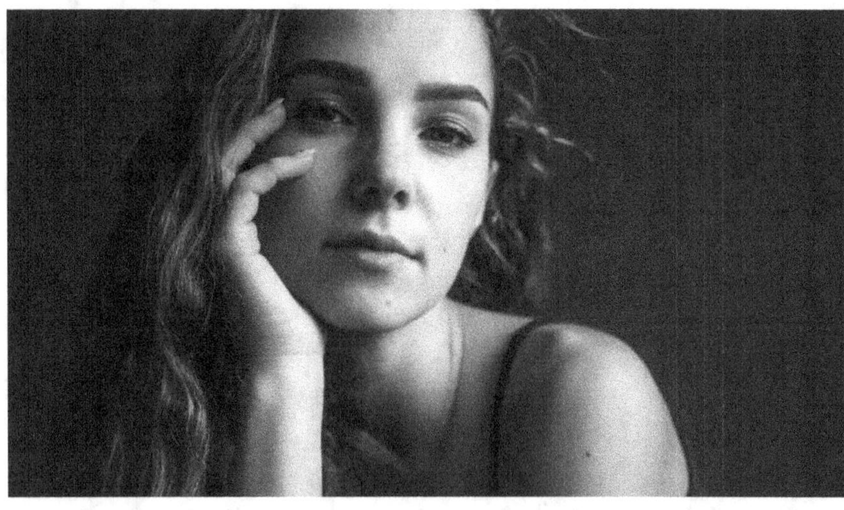

As we traverse the intricate landscape of midlife, the interconnectedness of body and mind becomes increasingly evident, especially during the transformative phase of menopause. It is a period that often heralds profound changes, not just physically but emotionally and mentally as well. Within this chapter, we explore the holistic approach to health, emphasizing how nurturing both the body and the mind can significantly enhance our well-being during this pivotal stage of life.

Menopause, often referred to as the 'second spring,' is a natural transition that every woman undergoes, yet its impact can be as unique as the women who experience it. To navigate this journey with grace and resilience requires an understanding that our physical health is deeply intertwined with our emotional state. As the ancient wisdom goes, 'A healthy outside starts from the inside.' This adage serves as a guiding principle throughout this chapter, reminding us that holistic health begins with nourishing our inner selves.

Scientific research has long established the significant role that physical health plays in influencing our mental and emotional well-being. During menopause, hormonal fluctuations can lead to a variety of symptoms, including mood swings, anxiety, and depression. However, studies have shown that lifestyle factors such as diet, exercise, and sleep can profoundly affect these symptoms, providing a natural way to mitigate their impact. By adopting a holistic approach, women can empower themselves to embrace menopause as an opportunity for growth and transformation rather than a period of decline.

Consider, for instance, the role of nutrition. A balanced diet rich in whole foods, particularly those high in phytoestrogens like flaxseeds and soy, can help manage menopausal symptoms by mimicking oestrogen in the body. Additionally, incorporating foods high in calcium and vitamin D supports bone health, which is crucial during this time. Through mindful eating, we can foster a sense of control and well-being that transcends mere physical nourishment, positively impacting our emotional state as well.

Exercise, too, plays a vital role in holistic health. Regular physical activity not only helps to manage weight and improve cardiovascular health but also acts as a natural mood booster by releasing endorphins, the body's feel-good hormones. Whether it's a brisk walk in nature, a yoga session, or a dance class, movement can be a powerful tool for fostering emotional balance and mental clarity.

Moreover, the importance of sleep cannot be overstated. Quality sleep is essential for both physical restoration and emotional regulation. Yet, many women find that menopause disrupts their sleep patterns, leading to fatigue and irritability. Implementing good sleep hygiene practices, such as establishing a regular bedtime routine and creating a restful sleep environment, can significantly improve sleep quality and, in turn, enhance overall well-being.

As we delve deeper into this chapter, the focus will be on practical strategies and tips that women can incorporate into their daily lives to nurture their body and mind. By embracing a holistic approach, we can transform the challenges of midlife into opportunities for renewed vitality and self-discovery. This journey toward holistic health is not just about enduring menopause but thriving through it, discovering the strength and wisdom that lies within us.

Ultimately, 'Body and Mind: Embracing Holistic Health' is an invitation to reimagine what wellness looks like during midlife, to see it not as a series of disjointed parts, but as an integrated whole. By aligning our physical health with our emotional and mental well-being, we create a harmonious balance that supports us through the transformative journey of menopause and beyond.

9.1 The Symphony of Body and Mind: Harmonizing Health in Menopause

The Resonance of Change

As women approach the threshold of menopause, a profound symphony begins to play — a harmonious blend of physical and emotional transformations. This life stage, often marked by a series of complex biological changes, invites us to explore a deeper connection between the body and mind, unveiling the intricate ways they influence each other. Understanding this connection is crucial in navigating the emotional waves that accompany menopause, empowering women to embrace a holistic approach to health.

The Biological Overture

Menopause is a natural biological process characterized by the cessation of menstruation and a decline in reproductive hormones such as oestrogen and progesterone. These hormonal shifts trigger a cascade of physical changes, including hot flashes, night sweats, and changes in metabolism. However, the impact of these fluctuations extends beyond the physical domain, deeply affecting emotional well-being. Research has shown that the decline in oestrogen levels can influence neurotransmitter activity in the brain, often leading to mood swings, anxiety, and depression.

This biological overture is not just a series of isolated events but a symphony that requires careful attention and understanding. By acknowledging the interplay between physical health and emotional states, women can better navigate the challenges of menopause and harness the transformative potential of this life stage.

Emotional Crescendos and Physical Echoes

The emotional crescendos experienced during menopause can manifest in various ways, from heightened sensitivity to stress to a newfound introspection and reflection. These emotional shifts are often mirrored in the body's responses, creating a feedback loop where physical symptoms can exacerbate emotional distress and vice versa.

For instance, sleep disturbances caused by night sweats can lead to fatigue and irritability, further impacting emotional resilience. Conversely, managing stress and cultivating emotional well-being can help alleviate some physical symptoms, fostering a sense of balance and harmony.

Embracing Mind-Body Practices

To navigate the intricate dance between body and mind, embracing mind-body practices becomes essential. Techniques such as mindfulness meditation, yoga, and tai chi offer powerful tools for cultivating awareness and reducing stress. By focusing on the present moment and fostering a non-judgmental attitude towards one's experiences, women can develop greater resilience and emotional regulation.

Mindfulness meditation, in particular, has been shown to reduce symptoms of anxiety and depression, improve sleep quality, and enhance overall well-being. Yoga and tai chi, with their emphasis on gentle movement and breath awareness, not only promote physical flexibility and strength but also encourage a deeper connection with the self.

Nourishing the Body and Mind

In addition to mind-body practices, nourishing the body with a balanced diet is crucial in maintaining emotional well-being during menopause. A diet rich in whole foods, including fruits, vegetables, lean proteins, and healthy fats, provides essential nutrients that support brain health and hormonal balance.

Particularly important are omega-3 fatty acids, found in fatty fish and flaxseeds, which have been linked to improved mood and cognitive function. Additionally, foods rich in phytoestrogens, such as soy products and flaxseeds, may help mitigate some menopausal symptoms by mimicking the effects of oestrogen in the body.

Hydration is another key component of physical and emotional health, as dehydration can contribute to fatigue and mood disturbances. Ensuring adequate water intake supports overall bodily functions and helps maintain energy levels.

The Wisdom of Rest and Recovery

In the symphony of body and mind, rest and recovery play a pivotal role. Prioritizing quality sleep is essential for emotional resilience and cognitive function, as the brain processes emotions and memories during restful slumber. Creating a sleep-friendly environment, maintaining a consistent sleep schedule, and practicing relaxation techniques before bedtime can enhance sleep quality.

Additionally, incorporating periods of rest and relaxation throughout the day allows the body and mind to rejuvenate, reducing stress and promoting a sense of calm. Activities such as reading, journaling, or simply spending time in nature can provide moments of tranquillity and reflection.

The Proverbial Wisdom of Harmony

As we explore the symphony of body and mind, the ancient proverb, "A sound mind in a sound body," offers profound wisdom. This timeless insight reminds us that nurturing both our physical and emotional selves is essential for holistic health. By embracing this interconnectedness, women can navigate the challenges of menopause with grace and resilience, uncovering new strengths and possibilities.

Conclusion: Embracing the Symphony

The journey through menopause is not merely a biological transition but an opportunity for profound growth and transformation. By recognizing and honouring the intricate connection between body and mind, women can embrace a holistic approach to health that nurtures both physical and emotional well-being.

In this symphony of change, each note—whether it be a physical symptom or an emotional wave—contributes to the rich tapestry of midlife. Through mindful practices, nourishing choices, and the wisdom of rest, women can harmonize their health and navigate this life stage with confidence and empowerment. As we embrace the symphony of body and mind, we discover the beauty and strength that lie within the dance of menopause, transforming solitude into a powerful catalyst for self-discovery and renewal.

9.2 Nourishing the Body, Nurturing the Mind: A Holistic Approach to Health

The Symphony of Nutrition: Fuelling Your Midlife Vitality

In the tapestry of life, food is a thread that weaves through our days, offering not only sustenance but also a reflection of our values and self-care. As women transition through midlife, the role of nutrition becomes increasingly paramount, serving as both a fuel for the body and a balm for the mind. During menopause, hormonal fluctuations can lead to various changes in metabolism, energy levels, and mood. It is here that a strategic approach to nutrition can serve as a powerful ally, transforming potential challenges into opportunities for renewed vitality.

Embracing Nutrient-Dense Foods

Nutrient density is key to maintaining energy and health during midlife. Foods rich in vitamins, minerals, and antioxidants can help combat the oxidative stress and inflammation often associated with aging and hormonal changes. Leafy greens, vibrant fruits, nuts, seeds, and whole grains are not merely ingredients but potent allies in the pursuit of wellness. Incorporating a variety of these foods ensures that your body receives the comprehensive nourishment it needs to thrive. For instance, calcium and vitamin D are crucial for maintaining bone health, while omega-3 fatty acids found in fish like salmon can support heart health and cognitive function.

Hydration: The Unsung Hero

Water is often overlooked in the conversation about nutrition, yet it plays a vital role in every aspect of health. Proper hydration supports digestion, aids in nutrient absorption, and helps regulate body temperature. For women experiencing menopause, staying hydrated can also help alleviate common symptoms such as hot flashes and headaches. Aiming for at least eight glasses of water a day, or more depending on individual needs, is a simple yet profound way to nurture both body and mind.

The Art of Mindful Eating

Mindful eating is a practice that encourages a deeper connection with food and the act of eating. By slowing down and savouring each bite, you not only enhance digestion but also create a moment of mindfulness that can reduce stress and improve your relationship with food. This practice invites you to listen to your body's hunger and fullness cues, fostering a more intuitive and nourishing approach to eating.

Moving with Purpose: Exercise for Body and Mind

Physical activity is a cornerstone of holistic health, offering benefits that extend far beyond the physical realm. For women in midlife, exercise becomes a vital tool for managing weight, improving mood, and maintaining strength and flexibility. The key is to find activities that bring joy and can be sustained over the long term, transforming exercise from a chore into a cherished part of daily life.

Strength Training: Building a Resilient Foundation

As we age, muscle mass naturally declines, which can affect metabolism and increase the risk of injury. Strength training is an effective way to counteract these changes, building muscle, enhancing bone density, and boosting metabolic rate. Activities like weightlifting, resistance band exercises, or bodyweight workouts can be tailored to individual fitness levels and incorporated into a balanced exercise routine. Not only does strength training fortify the body, but it also cultivates a sense of empowerment and resilience.

The Joy of Movement: Finding Your Passion

While structured exercise is important, finding joy in movement is equally essential. Whether it's dancing, hiking, swimming, or practicing yoga, engaging in activities that resonate with your interests can transform exercise into a source of pleasure and relaxation. This joyful movement not only supports physical health but also nurtures the mind, reducing stress and fostering a sense of happiness.

The Restorative Power of Sleep: Rejuvenating Body and Mind

Sleep is the body's natural reset button, a time when cells repair, memories consolidate, and the mind rejuvenates. Yet, for many women in midlife, sleep can become elusive, interrupted by night sweats, insomnia, or anxiety. Prioritizing quality sleep is essential for maintaining holistic health, affecting everything from metabolism to mood.

Creating a Sleep Sanctuary

The environment in which you sleep plays a significant role in the quality of rest you achieve. Transform your bedroom into a sleep sanctuary by keeping it cool, dark, and quiet. Consider investing in comfortable bedding and using blackout curtains to minimize light. Establishing a consistent bedtime routine, such as dimming lights, reading a calming book, or practicing relaxation techniques, can signal to your body that it's time to wind down.

The Role of Sleep Hygiene

Sleep hygiene encompasses the habits and practices that contribute to restorative sleep. Limiting caffeine and alcohol intake, especially in the hours leading up to bedtime, can prevent disruptions in sleep patterns. Similarly, reducing screen time and exposure to blue light from electronic devices can help regulate the body's natural sleep-wake cycle. Engaging in calming activities, such as meditation or gentle stretching, can further promote relaxation and ease the transition into sleep.

Balancing Body and Mind: The Path to Holistic Well-being

The journey to holistic health is one of balance, where nutrition, exercise, and sleep intertwine to support both body and mind. Embracing this trifecta of well-being allows you to navigate the complexities of midlife with grace and resilience. As you cultivate a deeper understanding of your body's needs and rhythms, you empower yourself to make choices that honour and nurture your whole being.

A Proverb for the Path Ahead

"Health is the greatest possession. Contentment is the greatest treasure. Confidence is the greatest friend." – Lao Tzu.

This ancient wisdom reminds us that true health encompasses more than the physical; it is a state of harmony and contentment that arises from within. By nurturing your body and mind through intentional nutrition, joyful movement, and restorative sleep, you cultivate a foundation of well-being that supports you in embracing the transformative journey of midlife solitude.

9.3 The Inner Symphony: Aligning Body and Mind

The Inner Symphony: Aligning Body and Mind

In the profound journey through midlife, the symbiotic relationship between body and mind becomes increasingly evident. The ancient wisdom, 'A healthy outside starts from the inside,' serves as a guiding principle, urging us to look beyond surface-level symptoms and embrace a holistic approach to health. This section explores the interconnectedness of our physical and mental well-being, emphasizing the importance of nurturing the mind to achieve a harmonious balance that radiates outward.

The Mind-Body Connection: An Ancient Understanding

For centuries, various cultures have recognized the interconnectedness of mind and body, a concept often overlooked in the hustle of modern life. Traditional Chinese Medicine, Ayurveda, and other ancient healing practices have long advocated for a holistic approach, suggesting that mental health directly influences physical health. Recent psychological research corroborates these ancient beliefs, revealing that stress, anxiety, and depression can manifest as physical ailments such as headaches, digestive issues, and chronic pain.

Understanding this interconnectedness is crucial, especially during menopause—a time when hormonal fluctuations can trigger both emotional and physical changes. Research indicates that women experiencing menopause are at a higher risk for mood disorders, which can exacerbate physical symptoms such as hot flashes and fatigue. By addressing mental health proactively, women can mitigate these impacts and foster a healthier, more resilient body.

Hormonal Changes: Navigating the Emotional Impact

The hormonal shifts during menopause significantly affect mood and cognitive function. Oestrogen, a hormone that plays a vital role in regulating mood and cognition, declines during menopause, leading to increased vulnerability to anxiety and depression. Studies have shown that the reduction of oestrogen can result in lower serotonin levels, a neurotransmitter critical for maintaining mood balance.

Despite these challenges, midlife offers an opportunity for introspection and self-awareness, allowing women to develop coping strategies that enhance mental resilience. Mindfulness practices such as meditation and yoga have been shown to improve mood and reduce stress levels, providing a buffer against the emotional turbulence of menopause.

Nurturing Mental Health: Strategies for Inner Well-being

1. Mindfulness and Meditation: Incorporating mindfulness into daily routines can significantly improve mental clarity and emotional stability. Research suggests that regular meditation practice can increase gray matter in the brain, enhancing cognitive function and emotional regulation. By dedicating time each day to mindfulness, women can cultivate a sense of calm and presence that supports overall well-being.

2. Cognitive Behavioural Therapy (CBT): CBT is a powerful tool for managing the negative thought patterns that often accompany menopause. By identifying and challenging these thoughts, women can develop healthier coping mechanisms and reduce symptoms of anxiety and depression. Studies have shown that CBT can be as effective as medication in treating mood disorders, with long-lasting benefits.

3. Social Support: Building and maintaining strong social connections is vital for mental health. Engaging with friends, family, or support groups can provide emotional support and reduce feelings of isolation. Research indicates that social interaction stimulates the production of oxytocin, a hormone that promotes feelings of trust and bonding, which can counteract the stress response.

Physical Health: The Reflection of Inner Balance

While mental health forms the foundation of well-being, physical health is its reflection. The body often mirrors the state of the mind, and by nurturing our mental health, we inevitably improve our physical condition.

1. Nutrition and Diet: A balanced diet rich in essential nutrients supports both physical and mental health. Omega-3 fatty acids, found in fish and flaxseeds, are known to enhance cognitive function and reduce inflammation. Similarly, antioxidants in fruits and vegetables protect against cellular damage and improve brain health. During menopause, maintaining a diet that balances blood sugar can alleviate mood swings and reduce the risk of developing chronic conditions such as diabetes.

2. Exercise and Physical Activity: Regular physical activity is a cornerstone of holistic health. Exercise releases endorphins, neurotransmitters that improve mood and reduce stress. Studies have shown that women who engage in regular physical activity experience fewer menopausal symptoms and have a lower risk of developing depression. Activities such as walking, swimming, and yoga not only enhance physical fitness but also provide mental clarity and emotional balance.

3. Sleep Hygiene: Quality sleep is essential for both physical and mental health. Hormonal changes during menopause can disrupt sleep patterns, leading to fatigue and irritability. Developing good sleep hygiene—such as maintaining a regular sleep schedule, creating a restful environment, and avoiding stimulants before bed—can improve sleep quality and overall well-being.

Embracing Holistic Health: A Lifestyle Approach

Holistic health is not a destination but a journey that requires continuous commitment and self-awareness. By understanding the interplay between mind and body, women can make informed choices that enhance their quality of life during midlife.

1. Self-Reflection and Goal Setting: Midlife is an ideal time for self-reflection and goal setting. By identifying personal values and aspirations, women can align their lifestyle choices with their inner desires, fostering a sense of purpose and fulfilment. This intentional living can enhance both mental and physical health, leading to a more balanced and satisfying life.

2. Integrative Therapies: Exploring integrative therapies such as acupuncture, massage, and aromatherapy can complement traditional medical treatments and support holistic health. These therapies can reduce

stress, alleviate physical symptoms, and promote relaxation, contributing to overall well-being.

3. Creative Expression: Engaging in creative activities such as art, music, or writing provides an outlet for self-expression and emotional release. Creative expression can enhance mood, increase self-awareness, and provide a sense of accomplishment and joy.

Conclusion: The Journey of Inner Harmony

Embracing holistic health during midlife requires a commitment to nurturing both the body and the mind. By acknowledging the intricate connection between mental and physical well-being, women can cultivate a lifestyle that supports resilience and vitality. The wisdom of 'A healthy outside starts from the inside' reminds us that true health emanates from within, and by nurturing our inner world, we can transform our outer reality. This journey of inner harmony not only enhances personal well-being but also empowers women to embrace the beauty and potential of midlife with grace and wisdom.

9.4 Embracing Holistic Health: A Path to Inner and Outer Well-Being

As we navigate the transformative journey of midlife, it becomes increasingly evident that the connection between our physical health and emotional well-being is profound and intricate, especially during menopause. By prioritizing our health holistically, we can foster resilience, vitality, and a deeper sense of peace. The wisdom that 'a healthy outside starts from the inside' resonates deeply here, reminding us that nurturing our inner selves is essential for external well-being. Key takeaways from this chapter include the importance of balanced nutrition, regular exercise, and restful sleep as foundational pillars of health. Consuming nutrient-rich foods can provide the energy and nutrients needed to support both body and mind. Engaging in activities that invigorate the body, whether through gentle exercises like yoga or brisk walks, enhances physical strength and emotional equilibrium. Additionally, prioritizing quality sleep replenishes our bodies, sharpens our minds, and stabilizes our moods. By embracing these strategies, we open the door to a harmonious, healthier life, where the synergy between body and mind encourages a fulfilling and joyful existence. Let these insights guide you on your path to holistic health, empowering you to experience midlife with grace, strength, and serenity.

Chapter 9: Reflection Time

- How do you perceive the connection between your physical health and emotional well-being during menopause?
- What changes in nutrition, exercise, or sleep have made a positive impact on your overall health?

- Reflect on the wisdom about a healthy outside starting from the inside. How can you nurture this holistic approach?

CHAPTER 10

The Journey Forward: Embracing the Next Chapter of Your Life

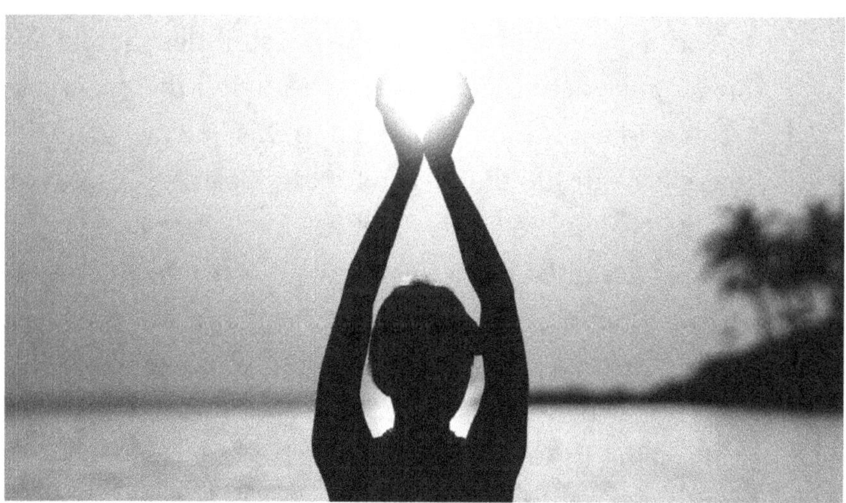

As you hold this book in your hands, you find yourself at the threshold of a new beginning, a journey forward into the uncharted territories of your life. The chapters you have traversed have equipped you with the wisdom and strategies needed to navigate the profound solitude that often accompanies midlife. Now, with a heart full of courage and a spirit brimming with optimism, you stand ready to embrace the future. This is a time not just to reflect but to act, to plant seeds for the years to come, even if the soil has been untouched for decades. As the ancient proverb wisely states, 'The best time to plant a tree was 20 years ago. The second best time is now.' This powerful reminder urges us to acknowledge that it's never too late to cultivate new dreams and aspirations.

Midlife is often painted as a period of decline, but in truth, it can be a time of rebirth and rejuvenation. This final chapter invites you to shed any remnants of doubt and to step boldly into a phase of life that promises growth and fulfilment. It encourages you to imagine the possibilities that lie ahead and to take active steps toward realizing them. Setting new goals and aspirations is crucial to this journey. Consider the areas of your life that yearn for attention and care. Perhaps it is time to explore a new hobby, travel to a place you've always dreamed of, or even embark on a new career path. Allow yourself to dream without constraints, knowing that each aspiration, no matter how grand or humble, is a testament to your resilience and your desire to thrive. Embracing the journey forward also involves cultivating a mindset of gratitude and presence.

Acknowledge the experiences that have shaped you, both the joyful and the challenging, and understand that they have contributed to the person you are today. Solitude in midlife has been a powerful teacher, revealing layers of strength and wisdom you may not have known you possessed. Now, as you look forward, let that wisdom guide you in making choices that align with your true self. This chapter is not merely a conclusion but a springboard into the future. It calls you to embrace change with open arms and to trust in the unfolding of your path. As you set out, remember that each step you take is a step toward greater understanding and fulfilment. The solitude you have embraced is not a lonely journey but a companion that has prepared you for this moment. This is your time—a time to plant, to nurture, and to watch the seeds of your dreams grow into reality. As you prepare to turn the page, take a deep breath and envision the horizon before you.

The journey forward is not just about where you will go, but who you will become along the way. Embrace this chapter with an open heart, and let the possibilities of the future inspire you. Remember, the journey is as important as the destination, and now, with newfound wisdom and strength, you are ready to embark on this exciting new chapter of your life.

10.1 Embracing the Horizon: Courage and Optimism for the Future

The Dawn of a New Chapter: Courage Unveiled

As we stand at the threshold of the next chapter in our lives, the future may appear as an expansive horizon, both daunting and exhilarating. Embracing this horizon requires the courage to step forward with optimism, a quality that can illuminate the path ahead, even when it seems shrouded in uncertainty. Courage, as ancient wisdom often reminds us, is not the absence of fear but the mastery of it. An old Cherokee proverb states, "The soul would have no rainbow if the eyes had no tears." This poignant reminder serves as a metaphor for the midlife transition, suggesting that the beauty of the next stage is born from the trials and experiences that precede it.

The Psychology Behind Optimism: A Scientific Perspective

Research in psychology reveals that optimism is not merely a sunny disposition but a powerful cognitive attribute that can be cultivated. According to a study published in the Journal of Personality and Social Psychology, optimism is linked to better health outcomes, increased resilience, and enhanced problem-solving skills. For women navigating the transformative phase of menopause, these benefits can be particularly impactful. The hormonal shifts and emotional changes can be challenging, yet by fostering an optimistic outlook, women can transform potential setbacks into opportunities for growth.

Optimism acts as a buffer against the stressors that accompany midlife changes. It encourages adaptive coping strategies, enhances social support networks, and fosters a sense of agency and control over one's life. In this way, optimism is not just a passive state of mind but an active approach to life's challenges, particularly during the midlife transition.

Finding Strength in Solitude: A Journey Inward

The journey of midlife solitude is not just a physical transformation but a profound psychological voyage. It is a time to rediscover and redefine oneself, to explore the depths of individuality that often go unnoticed amid the cacophony of daily responsibilities. Solitude offers a sanctuary—a space free from external judgments where one can reconnect with inner strengths and personal values.

Consider the wisdom of the poet Rainer Maria Rilke, who once said, "The only journey is the one within." This sentiment resonates deeply with the experience of midlife solitude, where the inner voyage becomes a source of empowerment. By embracing solitude, women can unearth hidden talents, reignite passions, and cultivate a resilient spirit capable of facing the future with renewed vigour.

Building a Vision for the Future: Crafting a Personal Narrative

A pivotal aspect of embracing the future is crafting a personal narrative that reflects one's values, aspirations, and sense of purpose. This narrative acts as a guiding star, providing clarity and direction amid the complexities of life. As women navigate menopause and the accompanying shifts, it becomes crucial to revisit and reframe their life stories.

The process of crafting this narrative involves reflecting on past experiences, acknowledging achievements, and identifying lessons learned. It also requires envisioning the future—not as a continuation of the past but as a canvas ripe with new possibilities. By articulating a personal narrative, women can align their actions with their core beliefs, paving the way for a meaningful and fulfilling future.

The Role of Community: Strength in Connection

While solitude can be a wellspring of personal growth, it is equally important to recognize the strength that comes from community and connection. Humans are inherently social creatures, and the bonds we form with others can provide support, encouragement, and a sense of belonging. As women embrace midlife, fostering meaningful relationships becomes a vital component of navigating the journey forward.

Building a community of like-minded individuals—whether through support groups, social clubs, or online platforms—can offer a network of understanding and empathy. These connections serve as reminders that the journey of midlife is shared and that collective wisdom can illuminate the path ahead. The African proverb "If you want to go fast, go alone. If you want to go far, go together" encapsulates the essence of community, underscoring the importance of unity and collaboration in achieving long-term goals.

Cultivating Resilience: The Heart of Optimism

Resilience, the ability to bounce back from adversity, is a key attribute that underpins optimism. It is the heart of embracing the future with courage and positivity. Resilience is not an innate trait but a skill that can be developed through intentional practices and mindsets.

To cultivate resilience, women can engage in activities that promote emotional well-being, such as mindfulness meditation, journaling, and physical exercise. These practices enhance emotional regulation, reduce stress, and foster a sense of inner peace. Moreover, adopting a growth mindset—believing in the ability to learn and grow through challenges—can reinforce resilience.

Embracing Change: An Invitation to Transformation

Change is an inevitable part of life, and midlife is often a period of significant transition. Instead of resisting change, women can view it as an invitation to transformation. This perspective shift allows for the acceptance of new realities and the exploration of uncharted territories.

Change can bring about a renaissance of self-discovery and reinvention. It is an opportunity to reassess priorities and pursue passions that may have been set aside. By embracing change, women can unlock their potential, uncover new talents, and experience the joy of lifelong learning.

Setting Intentions: Guiding Principles for the Future

To navigate the future with clarity and purpose, setting intentions can be a powerful tool. Intentions differ from goals in that they focus on the desired state of being rather than specific outcomes. They serve as guiding principles that shape daily actions and decisions.

For women in midlife, setting intentions might involve cultivating self-compassion, nurturing creativity, or prioritizing health and well-being. These intentions provide a framework for living authentically and aligning one's life with personal values. As intentions are set and acted upon, they create a ripple effect, influencing not only the individual but also the communities and environments they engage with.

Conclusion: The Path Ahead

The journey forward in midlife is a tapestry woven with threads of courage, optimism, and resilience. It is a time of profound transformation, offering the chance to redefine oneself and embrace the future with open arms. By cultivating optimism, crafting a personal narrative, building community, and setting intentions, women can navigate this transition with grace and wisdom.

In the words of the philosopher Lao Tzu, "A journey of a thousand miles begins with a single step." Let this be the guiding principle as you embark on the next chapter of life. With each step taken in courage and optimism, the path ahead becomes illuminated, revealing the boundless possibilities that await.

10.2 Charting New Horizons: Setting Goals for the Future

In the transformative journey of midlife solitude, the prospect of setting new goals and aspirations can seem daunting yet exhilarating. This period of life, often marked by the profound shifts of menopause, invites a re-evaluation of who we are and what we desire for our future. As the poet Mary Oliver wisely asked, 'Tell me, what is it you plan to do with your one wild and precious life?' This question becomes even more pertinent as we navigate the complexities and opportunities of midlife, a time ripe for reflection, reinvention, and revitalization.

The Canvas of Possibilities

Midlife is not simply an endpoint or a time of winding down but rather a canvas of possibilities waiting to be explored. It is an invitation to dream anew, to articulate aspirations that align with our evolved selves. The psychological concept of 'possible selves' comes into play here. This theory suggests that envisioning different versions of ourselves can guide behaviour and motivate change. By conceptualizing the person we wish to become, we can set concrete, actionable goals that steer us toward that vision.

For women experiencing the unique challenges and transitions of menopause, setting new goals can be both a coping mechanism and a pathway to empowerment. Imagine the possibilities: pursuing a long-held passion, embarking on a new career path, or dedicating time to personal growth and learning. Each goal represents a brushstroke on the vast canvas of your future, contributing to a masterpiece that is uniquely yours.

Goal-Setting: A Psychological Perspective

Psychologically, goal-setting plays a crucial role in well-being. Research has shown that individuals who set specific and challenging goals are more likely to achieve them and report higher levels of satisfaction and happiness. This is particularly relevant during midlife, as it is a phase characterized by substantial shifts in identity and purpose.

The SMART model — specific, measurable, achievable, relevant, and time-bound — offers a practical framework for goal-setting. By ensuring that goals are clearly defined and realistic, women in midlife can harness their inner resources and external support systems to achieve them. This structured approach provides clarity and direction, reducing the ambiguity that often accompanies periods of transition.

Moreover, the act of setting goals can mitigate feelings of loneliness and isolation. It fosters a sense of agency and control, empowering women to navigate their journeys with confidence and resilience. As you contemplate your aspirations, consider how they align with your values and passions. Let them be a beacon, guiding you through the complexities of midlife toward a future rich with purpose and fulfilment.

Embracing Change: The Role of Adaptability

The journey of setting new goals in midlife is intrinsically linked to adaptability. As we age, the ability to embrace change becomes an invaluable asset. The process of goal-setting itself requires flexibility — the understanding that goals may need to evolve as circumstances change.

Menopause is a period of significant biological and psychological transformation. It can be a time of profound introspection, prompting questions about identity and life direction. Embracing this change involves recognizing the strengths and wisdom accumulated over the years and using them as a foundation to build upon.

The ancient Chinese philosopher Lao Tzu famously said, 'When I let go of what I am, I become what I might be.' This wisdom highlights the importance of releasing past identities that no longer serve us, making space for new possibilities. By adopting a mindset of adaptability, women in midlife can navigate the inevitable ebbs and flows of life, staying focused on their goals while remaining open to new opportunities.

The Intersection of Solitude and Aspirations

Solitude, often perceived as loneliness, is reframed as a powerful catalyst for goal-setting in midlife. In the quiet moments of reflection, free from the distractions of the outside world, women can connect with their inner selves and discern what truly matters.

Research in positive psychology underscores the benefits of solitude in fostering creativity and self-awareness. It is in these moments of introspection that new ideas and aspirations can emerge, unfiltered by external expectations. By embracing solitude, women can cultivate a deeper understanding of their desires and motivations, paving the way for meaningful goal-setting.

Moreover, solitude offers an opportunity to assess past achievements and challenges. It is a time to honour the journey that has brought you to this moment, recognizing the resilience and strength that have carried you through. As you contemplate your future, let solitude be a companion, offering clarity and insight into the goals that will shape the next chapter of your life.

Building a Supportive Environment

While solitude is a powerful tool for self-discovery, the journey of setting and achieving new goals is often enriched by the support of others. Building a network of encouragement and accountability can enhance motivation and perseverance.

Social connections play a vital role in maintaining well-being throughout life. For women in midlife, fostering relationships with like-minded individuals who share similar aspirations can be particularly rewarding. Consider joining groups or communities that align with your interests, where you can exchange ideas and support one another's journeys.

Mentorship is another valuable resource. Seeking guidance from those who have walked similar paths can provide insights and inspiration, helping to navigate potential obstacles. Whether through formal mentorship programs or informal relationships, the wisdom of others can illuminate your path and reinforce your commitment to your goals.

Nurturing Holistic Well-being

As you set new goals for the future, it is essential to consider the holistic well-being of body and mind. Physical health, mental clarity, and emotional balance are interconnected facets that influence your ability to pursue and achieve your aspirations.

Engage in practices that nurture your well-being, such as regular exercise, meditation, and mindfulness. These activities not only enhance physical health but also promote mental clarity and emotional resilience. By prioritizing self-care, you create a solid foundation upon which to build your goals, ensuring that you have the energy and motivation to pursue them.

Moreover, adopting a growth mindset can be transformative. Embrace challenges as opportunities for learning and growth, viewing setbacks as stepping stones rather than obstacles. This perspective empowers you to persevere in the face of adversity, maintaining focus on your aspirations despite the inevitable ups and downs of life.

Crafting a Legacy

As you embark on the journey of setting new goals in midlife, consider the legacy you wish to leave behind. What impact do you want to have on the world, your community, and your loved ones? This reflection can provide profound motivation, imbuing your goals with a sense of purpose and meaning.

Legacy is not solely about grand achievements; it is also about the values and experiences you impart to others. Reflect on the qualities and lessons you hope to pass on, whether through mentorship, storytelling, or acts of kindness. By aligning your goals with your desired legacy, you create a roadmap that not only fulfils your personal aspirations but also contributes to the greater good.

A New Chapter Awaits

As you stand at the threshold of this new chapter in your life, the possibilities are as vast as the horizon. Embrace the journey with curiosity and courage, setting goals that reflect your deepest desires and values. Remember, midlife is not an ending but a beginning—a time to rediscover passions, redefine identity, and reimagine the future.

In the words of the renowned author and mythologist Joseph Campbell, 'We must be willing to let go of the life we planned so as to have the life that is waiting for us.' Allow this sentiment to guide you as you set forth on your journey, trusting that each step brings you closer to a life rich with fulfilment and purpose. Let your goals be the compass that directs your path, leading you toward the bright and promising future that awaits.

10.3 The Seeds of Tomorrow: Embracing New Beginnings

Cultivating the Garden of Life

As we journey through the passage of midlife, the landscape of our lives can often feel like an untended garden. We may find ourselves surrounded by the remnants of past seasons, with their faded blooms and scattered seeds. However, this is not a time to lament what once was, but rather an opportunity to cultivate something new. The proverb, 'The best time to plant a tree was 20 years ago. The second best time is now,' reminds us that it is never too late to sow the seeds of change and growth.

In the context of midlife solitude, this wisdom is particularly poignant. Menopause, with its profound physical and emotional shifts, can often feel like a storm that sweeps through our lives, leaving us in silence. Yet, this silence is fertile ground; it is a chance to plant the seeds of our future selves, to nurture the dreams and aspirations that might have been overshadowed by the busyness of earlier years.

Understanding the Soil: The Psychological Landscape

Before we can plant new seeds, we must first understand the soil in which they will grow. The psychological landscape of midlife solitude is complex, shaped by experiences of loneliness, transformation, and introspection. Research in the field of psychology reveals that loneliness can have significant impacts on mental health, particularly for women over 50 who are navigating menopause. Studies suggest that loneliness can exacerbate symptoms such as anxiety and depression, creating a cycle that is hard to break.

However, understanding these challenges is the first step in overcoming them. By acknowledging the presence of loneliness and the unique psychological shifts that accompany menopause, women can begin to prepare the soil of their minds for new growth. This involves cultivating self-awareness and compassion, recognizing that solitude is not a void to be filled, but a space to be embraced.

Planting the Seeds: New Beginnings in Solitude

With the soil prepared, it is time to plant the seeds of new beginnings. This process requires both courage and patience, as we learn to listen to the whispers of our hearts and to honour our deepest desires. For many women, midlife is a time of rediscovery and reinvention. It is an opportunity to explore passions that may have been set aside, to pursue new goals, and to redefine what success means.

Consider the story of Julia, a 55-year-old woman who found herself feeling unanchored as she entered menopause. Her children had left home, and she had retired from a long career that had defined much of her identity. Instead of succumbing to the loneliness that threatened to engulf her, Julia decided to embrace this new chapter. She enrolled in art classes and began painting, something she had always loved but never had time for. Through this creative expression, Julia found a sense of purpose and joy that reinvigorated her spirit.

Nurturing Growth: Patience and Perseverance

Once the seeds are planted, they must be nurtured with care and attention. Growth takes time, and it is important to be patient with ourselves as we navigate this journey. Menopause is a process, not an event, and the changes it brings unfold gradually. Similarly, the transformation that occurs in solitude is not immediate; it requires perseverance and a willingness to embrace the unknown.

Nurturing growth also involves tending to our emotional and physical well-being. This means prioritizing self-care, seeking support when needed, and allowing ourselves the grace to rest and recharge. Engaging in practices such as mindfulness, meditation, or yoga can help cultivate a sense of inner peace and resilience, providing the nourishment needed for our seeds of change to flourish.

Harvesting the Fruits: Embracing the Future

Eventually, the seeds we have planted begin to bear fruit. The dreams and goals that once seemed distant become tangible realities, and the solitude that once felt daunting transforms into a source of strength. This is the harvest of our journey forward, the culmination of our efforts to embrace the next chapter of our lives with grace and wisdom.

As we gather the fruits of our labour, we must also reflect on the journey that brought us here. Each step, each challenge, and each moment of solitude has contributed to our growth and transformation. By recognizing the power and resilience within us, we can move forward with confidence, ready to face whatever the future holds.

Continuing the Cycle: Planting Again

The journey of life is cyclical, and as we embrace the next chapter, we are reminded that each ending is also a new beginning. The seeds we plant today will shape the landscape of our future, and the choices we make now will influence the legacy we leave behind.

As we continue to plant and nurture new seeds, we are called to share our wisdom and experiences with others. By doing so, we become beacons of hope and inspiration, lighting the way for those who follow in our footsteps. In this way, the journey forward is not only a personal transformation but a collective one, as we contribute to a world that values and celebrates the beauty of midlife solitude.

Conclusion: The Journey Forward

As we conclude this exploration of midlife solitude, we are reminded that the journey forward is one of endless possibilities. The proverb, 'The best time to plant a tree was 20 years ago. The second best time is now,' serves as a powerful reminder that it is never too late to embrace change and growth. Through solitude, we find the strength to redefine our identities, to pursue our passions, and to build meaningful connections. Let us embrace this journey with open hearts and minds, ready to plant the seeds of our future and to cultivate the garden of our lives.

10.4 Embracing the Path Ahead

As you stand on the threshold of this new chapter in your life, remember to greet the future with optimism and courage. Each day offers a fresh canvas upon which to paint your aspirations and realize your potential. Setting new goals and nurturing your dreams are not merely tasks but a testament to your commitment to growth and self-discovery.

The proverb, 'The best time to plant a tree was 20 years ago. The second best time is now,' serves as a reminder that it is never too late to embark on new ventures. The seeds you plant today will become the foundation for a flourishing tomorrow. Whether it is pursuing a long-held passion, cultivating new relationships, or simply learning to savour the quiet moments, each step forward is an opportunity to enrich your life's journey.

In summary, embrace the possibilities that lie ahead with an open heart and a willing spirit. Let optimism guide you, and allow courage to propel you. Set clear, achievable goals that align with your values and aspirations. As you move forward, remember that every moment is ripe with potential, waiting to be transformed into a stepping stone along your path. With these reflections in mind, you are well-equipped to navigate the years to come with grace and purpose.

Chapter 10: Reflection Time

- What new goals and aspirations do you have for the coming years, and how do you plan to pursue them?
- How can you embrace the future with optimism and courage, despite any uncertainties?
- Reflect on the proverb about planting a tree. What actions can you take now to cultivate a fulfilling future?

CONCLUSION OF QUIET REFLECTIONS: WISDOM AND STRATEGIES FOR MIDLIFE SOLITUDE

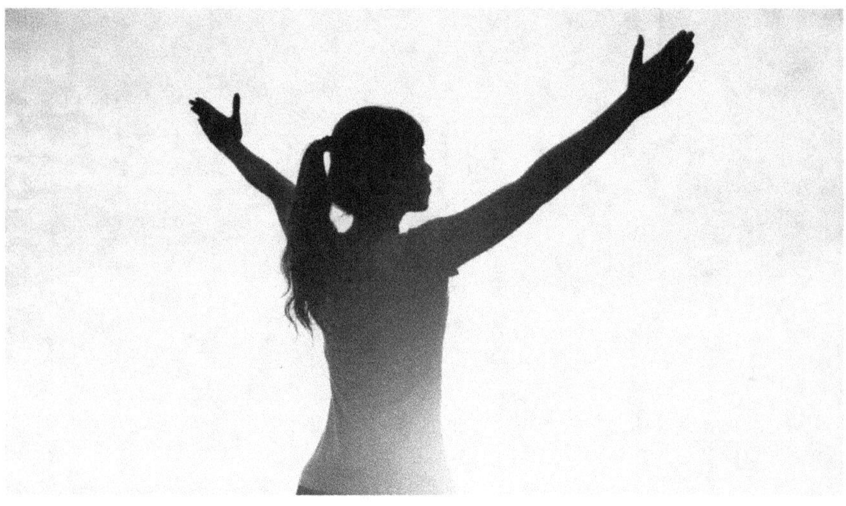

As we draw the curtains on 'Quiet Reflections: Wisdom and Strategies for Midlife Solitude,' let us take a moment to revisit the transformative journey we've embarked upon together. Throughout the chapters, we've explored the intricate dance between loneliness and solitude, uncovering the profound opportunities for growth and self-discovery that midlife presents.

In this book, we began by understanding the silent transition into midlife solitude, emphasizing the psychological perspectives on loneliness. We recognized the importance of embracing solitude as a gateway to self-discovery and redefined our identities amidst life's changes. Building resilience became a central theme, equipping us with the inner strength needed to navigate this unique phase.

We also explored the essential role of social connections and the power of finding purpose, all while managing the emotional waves that accompany midlife. With a focus on holistic health, we acknowledged the interconnectedness of body and mind, reinforcing the importance of nurturing both.

As you stand at this juncture, poised to embrace your solitude with newfound wisdom, consider these actionable steps:

1. Reflect and Reframe: Regularly set aside time for introspection. Use journaling or meditation to explore your thoughts and emotions, reframing solitude as an empowering ally rather than an isolating force.

2. Cultivate Connections: While solitude is valuable, human connections remain vital. Foster relationships that enrich your life, and don't hesitate to seek support when needed.

3. Pursue Purpose: Identify activities or causes that resonate with your values and passions. Engaging in purposeful endeavours can infuse your solitude with meaning and direction.

4. Prioritize Holistic Health: Take a holistic approach to your well-being by balancing physical activity, mental stimulation, and relaxation. Consider integrating practices like yoga, tai chi, or mindfulness into your routine.

5. Embrace Change: View the changes that accompany midlife as opportunities for growth. Welcome new experiences and challenges, allowing them to shape and refine your evolving identity.

In conclusion, midlife solitude is not merely a passage to endure; it is a profound opportunity to rediscover and reinvent yourself. As you continue on this path, remember that solitude, like a quiet lake, reflects the depth and beauty within you. May the wisdom and strategies shared in this book serve as a guiding light, helping you navigate this journey with grace, strength, and resilience.

MENOPAUSE RELIEF THERAPY

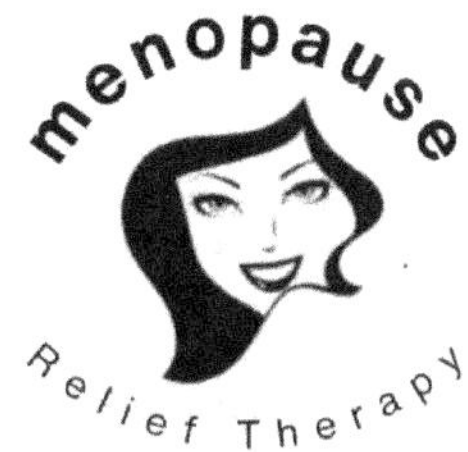

Resources

- Blog for Menopause Relief
  https://menopauserelieftherapy.co.uk/blog

- CBT (Cognitive Behavioural Therapy) Online
  Course for Menopause Hot Flushes Management
  https://cbt.selfhelpmenopausecourses.com

- Facebook
  https://www.facebook.com/MenopauseReliefTher
  apyForEmotionalWellbeing

- Instagram
  https://www.instagram.com/menopausereliefthera
  py

- Self-Help Courses for Menopause Relief
  https://members.selfhelpmenopausecourses.com

- TikTok
  https://www.tiktok.com/@menopause_relief_thera
  py

- YouTube Channel
  https://www.youtube.com/@menopausereliefthera
  py for Menopause Relief Strategies, Menopause Self-
  Care Tips, Menopause Affirmations, Menopause
  Meditations, Menopause Hypnotherapy for Hot
  Flushes and Menopause Psychoeducation

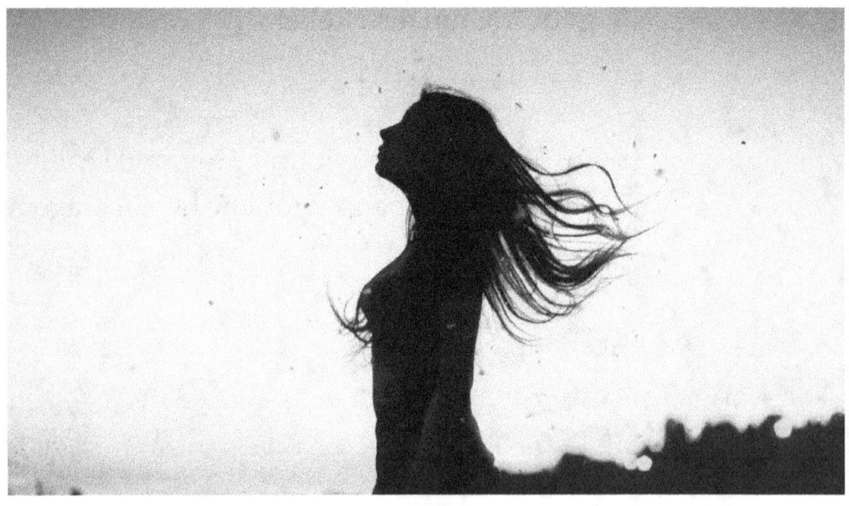